Also by C.W. Randolph, Jr., M.D.

and Genie James, M.M.Sc

From Belly Fat to Belly Flat

from Hormone HELL to Hormone WELL

Straight Talk Women (and Men) Need to Know to Save Their Sanity, Health, and—Quite Possibly—Their Lives

C.W. Randolph, Jr., M.D.
and Genie James, M.M.Sc
authors of *From Belly Fat to Belly Flat*

Health Communications, Inc.
Deerfield Beach, Florida

www.hcibooks.com

Library of Congress Cataloging-in-Publication Data

Randolph, C. W.
From hormone hell to hormone well : straight talk women (and men) need to know to save their sanity, health, and quite possibly their lives / C.W. Randolph Jr. and Genie James.
p. cm.
Includes bibliographical references and index.
ISBN-13: 978-0-7573-1390-5 (trade paper)
ISBN-10: 0-7573-1390-6 (trade paper)
1. Menopause—Hormone therapy. 2. Hormone therapy.
I. James, Genie. II. Title.
RG186.R36 2008
618.1'75061—dc22

2008049571

ISBN-13: 978-0-7573-1390-5
ISBN-10: 0-7573-1390-6

Publisher: Health Communications, Inc.
3201 S.W. 15th Street
Deerfield Beach, FL 33442-8190

Cover design by Larissa Hise Henoch
Inside book design and formatting by Dawn Von Strolley Grove

This book is dedicated to two courageous pioneers in the realm of hormone health. The first is the late John R. Lee, M.D. Dr. Lee committed his life's work to increasing awareness about the safety and efficacy of bio-identical hormone replacement therapies (BHRT) as an alternative to synthetic hormone replacement therapy. His ground-breaking book series, beginning with What Your Doctor May Not Tell You About Menopause, *continues his mission today. Dr. Lee's professional mentoring and personal friendship have left lasting fingerprints on my life and my medical practice.*

Next, Genie and I would like this book to honor the memory of Barbara Seaman, author of the seminal books The Doctor's Case Against the Pill *and* The Greatest Experiment Ever Performed on Women: Exploding the Estrogen Myth. *Though we never met Ms. Seaman before she passed in 2008, Genie communicated with her often. Like Dr. Lee, Ms. Seaman started a revolution in women's health by questioning what was being taken for granted and meticulously exposing the potentially carcinogenic effects of synthetic hormones.*

God bless,
C. W. Randolph, Jr., M. D.

Contents

4 The Truth About Male Menopause

5 It's Not Just Your Age . . . It's Your Life

6 More Than Uncomfortable: How Hormone Imbalance Impacts Health and Mortality

PART 3

THREE STEPS TO FEEL—AND LOOK—YOUNGER AND BETTER

APPENDIX: RESOURCE LISTING
GETTING HELP WHEN AND WHERE YOU NEED IT

Acknowledgments

There are many people to thank for their participation in moving this book from an idea to a work of art in print. First and foremost, I want to thank God for giving me the ability, knowledge, and talent to become a physician and healer. I am also privileged to be in a profession where I can actively serve as an instrument of my creator.

Second, I would like to thank my coauthor (and now wife) Genie James for her spiritual presence on every page of this book. I am grateful for her knowledge, drive, research, and ability to move fluidly from medical terminology to patient testimonies. I know that Genie's input helped us craft this book with language and tone that should have meaning both for healthcare professionals and consumers.

While I dedicated this book to John R. Lee, M.D., it is important for me to take this opportunity to underscore the seminal role he played in opening my mind and eyes to the clinical efficacy and safety of bio-identical hormone replacement. I also want to acknowledge Virginia Hopkins for her pivotal role in working with Dr. Lee to coauthor three books that have helped set the stage for the current revolution supporting the use of bio-identical hormone therapies: *What Your Doctor May Not Tell You About Pre-Menopause, What Your Doctor May Not Tell You About Menopause, and What Your Doctor May Not Tell You About Breast Cancer.*

Over the last few decades, there has been a groundswell of medical research validating the safety and efficacy of BHRT. It had been my privilege to dialogue frequently with several medical research pioneers. Specifically, I want to acknowledge Joel Hargrove, M.D., for his groundbreaking research on bio-identical progesterone therapy while serving as a clinical professor for the Department of Gynecologic Reproductive Endocrinology at Vanderbilt University's School of Medicine; Helene Leonetti, M.D., for her daring research on the clinical benefits of bio-identical progesterone cream; Kenna Stephenson, M.D., for her research validating bio-identical hormones as an effective and safe clinical therapy for women suffering from menopausal symptoms; and David Zava, Ph.D., for his research on bio-identical hormone replacement and breast cancer. I also want to express my gratitude to Carl Burak, M.D., for first introducing me to Dr. John Lee's work. Also, I want to thank his wife and my friend Ronnie Burak for her ever-encouraging words regarding my life's work and professional direction.

My appreciation for our team of experts at Health Communications Inc. (HCI) is without bounds. Special thanks are due to our editors Allison Janse and Michelle Matrisciani. In addition, this book has legs because of the superior marketing and public relations skills of Nannette Noffsinger, our personal media and public relations consultant, and Kim Weiss, marketing coordinator for HCI.

This book, and my mission, would not be possible without the medical, professional, and administrative staff of my Ageless and Wellness Medical Center. I continue to learn from and be in awe of their day-to-day willingness to, first, listen to our patients' concerns, and then to treat each individual with heartfelt compassion and respect.

Finally, I want to acknowledge my patients. This book would have no purpose or meaning without them, their clinical results, and their personal testimonies. My hope is that by sharing the stories of my patients who have benefited from the bio-identical treatment regimens described in this text, I can help millions of other women (and men) find their voices to demand that their hormone health be taken seriously.

Introduction

As a board-certified obstetrician and gynecologist (OB/GYN) working with a team of qualified and gifted medical professionals, my Ageless and Wellness Medical Center serves close to ten thousand patients—women and men—each year. My focus is hormone health, and my expertise is bio-identical hormone replacement therapy (BHRT). Today, I am humbled to be internationally recognized for my natural approach to treating the symptoms and health concerns that result from the aging body's shift in hormone production. But like most traditional physicians today, I did not always understand or prescribe BHRT for my patients.

Along with every other physician who graduated from medical school in the last several decades, I was trained to believe that synthetic hormone replacement therapy (HRT) provided a number of health benefits for women suffering from the symptoms of hormonal changes. The touted benefits of synthetic hormone replacement included relief from hot flashes and vaginal dryness, and preventing osteoporosis. Medical schools also taught that a complete hysterectomy (removing the uterus, tubes, and ovaries) was the recommended treatment for women with dysfunctional bleeding, fibroid tumors, or endometriosis with chronic pelvic pain. For years, leading women's health experts contended that—for a woman who had all the children she wanted or who was past childbearing age—the ovaries were just inert fibrous tissue masses that served no function for the aging female body. Today, I am convinced, and have the clinical evidence to prove, that the training we physicians received from our respective medical schools was dead wrong.

When I opened my practice in 1986, I initially adhered to my medical school training and regularly prescribed synthetic HRT, such as the pharmaceutical brands Premarin, Provera, and Prempro, for patients who had undergone a hysterectomy or who were suffering from menopausal symptoms. When asked about side effects, including weight gain or long-term health risks, I repeated what I had been taught: that there was no clinical evidence to support these concerns. Nevertheless, it took only a couple of years for me to seriously doubt my training when I saw what these synthetic hormones were doing to my patients.

Many of the women who began taking the prescribed synthetic HRT gained a great deal of weight that couldn't be attributed to changes in eating habits or lifestyle activities; the only thing that had changed for them was the introduction of synthetic estrogen into their bodies. In addition to their concerns about weight gain, these same patients frequently came in with new complaints including bloating, decreased libido, depression, poor quality of sleep, and "just not feeling right."

What I heard and observed confused me. I began to ask myself, if what I had been taught about HRT and weight gain could be wrong, what other aspects of my medical training regarding synthetic hormone replacement might be, too? I determined to take a deeper look.

First, I tested to see if my patients' responses validated what was then the accepted medical theory that HRT would help prevent osteoporosis. It didn't. When I tested the bone mineral density of my patients who had been on HRT, I found that instead of evidencing an increase in bone density, many had developed borderline or true osteoporosis! Suddenly my confusion turned to real concern. Was HRT helping or hurting my patients?

Finally, I became highly concerned about the potential correlation between synthetic HRT and my patients' breast health. I found that when I put women on synthetic HRT, they were likely to return six months to a year later with fibrocystic breasts. Even though the volume of patients I was personally tracking did not equate to a statistically sound research database, I saw enough to make me question whether the synthetic HRT I was prescribing for my patients was causing excessive breast cell proliferation or growth.

From that point on, my concerns regarding the potentially negative health concerns associated with synthetic HRT transmuted from confusion and concern to a mixture of fear and anger. Excessive cell proliferation is a known precursor to cancer. Were the synthetic hormones actually having a carcinogenic effect? And if the answer was yes, what could I do to protect my patients?

All of these questions came to a head for me in the

early 1990s, a decade before the traditional medical establishment began to question the safety and efficacy of synthetic HRT. Fortunately, I had been a compounding pharmacist before returning to medical school. My intensive background in pharmacology combined with an in-depth understanding of the molecular structure of hormones and their respective receptors accelerated my disillusionment as well as my search for alternatives. In the early stages of my research I came upon Dr. John Lee's first book, *Natural Progesterone: The Multiple Roles of a Remarkable Hormone*. With Dr. Lee's book as my compass, my research moved in a new direction. I discovered ample medical research supporting the safety and efficacy of bio-identical progesterone replacement therapy. With the medical science in hand, I began to prescribe and compound bio-identical progesterone for my patients suffering from hormone imbalances. The result was symptomatic relief without the side effects of health risks characteristic of synthetic hormone replacement.

Today there is a groundswell of paranoia regarding synthetic HRT as a choice for treating menopausal symptoms, as well as for the prevention of some postmenopausal conditions. These much-publicized concerns are primarily derived from the National Institutes of Health (NIH)–sponsored Women's Health Initiative (WHI) study released in 2002. The findings indicated that the women in the study on HRT evidenced an increased risk of heart disease, breast cancer, stroke, and blood clots.

More than ten years after I was dubbed a maverick for taking my patients off synthetic hormones, WHI validated my concerns and reported that synthetic HRT is most definitely dangerous and quite possibly lethal. Despite the clinical evidence of this large-scale federally funded study, the controversy and confusion about hormone replacement continues to rage. HRT is not only still on the market, but it remains the most commonly prescribed treatment for women suffering from symptoms of hormone imbalance.

How can this be true? It is all about money. Synthetic HRT continues to be the most recommended treatment for women complaining of menopausal symptoms because of the millions of dollars the pharmaceutical companies spend marketing to physicians in their offices and at medical conferences. Even more egregious than the brainwashing of physicians is the pharmaceutical industry's more recent efforts to mislead the everyday consumer via expensive advertising campaigns.

When marketing, illusion, and the desire for profit outpace medical science, people suffer. From my clinical experience treating tens of thousands of patients, as well as the output of decades of respected medical research, I know that BHRT is safe and effective.

Still, I don't want you to take my word for it any more than I want you to innocently buy into pharmaceutical advertising promises. My aim in writing this book is to expose the truth about hormone replacement options so that you can make informed choices. My larger hope is that after reading this book, you will never again let any medical expert or outside entity usurp responsibility for your personal health and well-being. Your body, your mind, and your life are your own. I urge you to take charge.

PART 1

Women Taking Control: Dismissing Marketing Hype, Demanding Medical Science

My guess is that you picked up this book because, over the last several years, you have experienced changes in your body, mind, and moods that disturb you. You have struggled with weight gain, depression, foggy thinking, or low sex drive and possibly suffered through hot flashes, night sweats, irregular bleeding, vaginal dryness, or changes in breast tissue. You believe that somehow your age and hormones (or lack thereof) are in collusion, and if you don't do something, you are doomed to be increasingly fat, snippy, sexless, and senile. You would consider hormone replacement therapy (HRT), but over the last several years you've read in the newspaper or heard on television that those once-popular drugs have been linked to an increased risk of breast and uterine cancers, heart attack, stroke, and Alzheimer's disease. Your question is: do I have another option?

The answer is a resounding "Yes!" Bio-identical hormone replacement therapy (BHRT) has been clinically proven to be a safe and effective alternative for treating symptoms of hormone imbalance. Even better, BHRT goes beyond the symptoms to replace hormone deficiencies and biochemically resolve the problem at a cellular level.

In chapter 1, you will read the history behind the launch and promotion of pharmaceutically manufactured synthetic hormones, promoted despite the early evidence of their health dangers. You will learn how corrupt pharmaceutical industry practices have kept synthetic hormones on the market, despite mounting medical evidence linking these drugs to lethal health concerns. Then, in chapter 2, you'll learn about bio-identical hormones: what they are, how they are made, why they can't be patented and—most eye-opening—why you (and your doctor) may not have heard of them before now.

1 Decades of Desperate Women Dangerously Duped

For decades, pharmaceutically manufactured synthetic hormone replacement therapies have been touted as the female fountain of youth. "Take this pill and you can maintain your youthful good looks, increase your sexual energy, and keep a positive outlook for life," doctors and advertisements told women. To boot, doctors were convinced that synthetic hormones could help aging women keep their hearts, bones, and brains healthy. But in recent years an unrelenting stream of medical evidence has indicted synthetic hormone replacement therapy as an evil of its own, raising a woman's risk of heart disease, breast and uterine cancers, blood clotting and strokes, and Alzheimer's disease.

When the health risks associated with synthetic hormones first became public knowledge, millions of women on these drugs (such as the commonly prescribed Premarin or Prempro) were horrified. Their doctors were surprised and confused. Not so the medical experts employed by the pharmaceutical giants manufacturing these dangerous drugs. They had been aware of medical research evidencing the carcinogenic properties of synthetic estrogen since the early 1940s.

The Auschwitz Connection

Some of the first scientific experiments with synthetic hormones were conducted at Auschwitz.[1] The lead researcher was Adolph Friedrich Johann Butenandt, a biochemist (sponsored by the Schering pharmaceutical company) who won a Nobel Prize in 1939 for isolating sex hormones. According to previously sealed files of Nazi-era science, Butenandt's work included the introduction of three synthetic hormone products: Progynon, a synthetic estrogen; Proluton, a synthetic progesterone, or progestin; and Testoviron, the synthetic male hormone. In sponsoring Butenandt's research, Schering's marketing goal was to identify a way of using synthetic hormones as a form of birth control.

Excerpts from primary source documents obtained from archives in England and Germany describe the sterilization experiments. Women in Auschwitz were unknowingly fed daily doses of synthetic estrogen in their rutabaga soup. The goal of these experiments was to sterilize non-Aryans. Though unable to reproduce, the Jews would still be able to work as slave laborers for the "superior" Aryan race.[2]

In 1972, Dr. Jean Jofen presented to the Fifth World Congress of Jewish Studies a paper titled "Long-Range Effects of Medical Experiments in Concentration Camps: The Effect of Administration of Estrogen to the Mother on the Intelligence of the Offspring." Jofen reported that, after testing hundreds of children of Holocaust survivors, the Auschwitz contingent had the lowest IQ range. Dr. Jofen postulated that the synthetic hormone experiments were responsible.[3]

The DES Story

Diethylstilbestrol (DES) was a synthetic hormone drug first synthesized in 1938 by Sir Charles Dodd. It was the first synthetic hormone product that was cheap to manufacture and effective to take by mouth. Originally marketed as a "synthetic compound capable of producing the feminization effect similar to that of naturally occurring estrogen," DES was commonly prescribed during pregnancy to prevent miscarriages or premature deliveries.

In the United States, an estimated 5 to 10 million people were exposed to DES from 1938 to 1971, including pregnant women prescribed DES and their children. Nine out of every ten daughters of women who took DES had deformed reproductive systems or other abnormalities. Half would never be able to conceive or bear children. One in seven DES daughters contracted a rare and often lethal form of cancer called adenocarcinoma. This malignancy affects glandular tissue that forms only in those women whose mothers took DES during their first months of pregnancy. DES was also linked to a relatively rare form of testicular cancer in sons.[4]

In 1971, the Food and Drug Administration (FDA)

advised physicians to stop prescribing DES. While DES was the first synthetic hormone product to be named a human carcinogen, unfortunately, it wouldn't be the last.

A Huge Cover-Up

The HRT cover-up is much bigger than most people think. For over forty years, women and their physicians have been getting bad information from the pharmaceutical industry, while the federal government has done little to intervene.

Synthetic hormones are chemically altered hormones synthesized in a laboratory to have a different molecular structure than the hormones produced by the ovaries or testes. Why wouldn't the pharmaceutical companies synthesize a hormone with exactly the same molecular structure as the ones produced by the body? Because you can't patent a molecular structure that occurs in nature. By altering the molecular structure of the hormones, the pharmaceutical manufacturer can have exclusive ownership of both the chemical formula and the revenue generated by its synthetic hormone product until its patent expires.

Synthetic Hormone Brand Names

Premarin	Combipatch
Prempro	Cenestin
Premphase	Menest
Femhrt	Orth-est
Activella	Ogen
Ortho-prefest	Estratab

Premarin, a synthetic estrogen made from the urine of pregnant mares, was put on the market by Ayerst Laboratories in 1942, just one year after a study published in the journal *Cancer Research* reported, "Estrogen is a very important factor, not merely an incidental one, in cervical carcinogenesis." How did the medical community overlook the output of this study? The answer, once again, is pharmaceutical marketing. Consider the dollars at stake.

The marketing launch of Premarin was aggressive and conspicuous. The consumer print ads took one of two approaches. The first was to feature glamorous, happy, and thin middle-aged women attributing their health, beauty, and vitality to their new hormone pill. In subsequent years the tone of the ads changed. Angry and disheveled middle-aged women loomed over captions like, "Is it *her*, or is it *her hormones*?" or "Do you really want to outlive your ovaries?"

In concert with the direct-to-consumer campaign, pharmaceutical sales representatives blazed trails into doctors' offices armed with lunch and marketing materials. They convinced doctors that these new synthetic hormones could eliminate their previous frustration of having limited success treating menopausal symptoms. Even better, these representatives purported, synthetic hormone replacement drugs would protect the bones and hearts of female patients.

What Is "Synthetic"

- *"Patented" or "Conventional" or "Artificial"*
- *Usually not found in nature or at least not in humans*
- *Chemically altered form of human hormone*
- *Not identical in structure or activity to natural hormones they try to emulate*

By the 1970s, Premarin was regarded as the gold standard for treating menopausal symptoms such as hot flashes, night sweats, vaginal dryness and atrophy, depression, mood swings, and low libido. For several years, the merged pharmaceutical giant Wyeth-Ayerst capitalized on the synthetic hormone market niche and relished its position as a leader in the women's health market. Then, in 1975, medical evidence caused the company to fumble. Clinical studies reported a link between the synthetic horse estrogen in Premarin and uterine (endometrial) cancer.

As a result of the clinical evidence, the FDA took its first stand on this issue. Wyeth-Ayerst was required to include a black-box warning as a package insert with every prescription. A black-box warning is the strongest type of warning that the FDA can require for a drug and is generally reserved for alerting patients to adverse drug reactions that can cause serious injury or death. Many medical researchers contended that the adverse reactions associated with Premarin were so significant that the FDA should have by-passed the black-box warning and immediately pulled the dangerous drug off the market.

The Official Black-Box Warning for Premarin

Important Safety Information

What is the most important information you should know about PREMARIN (estrogens), PREMPRO (a combination of estrogens and a progestin), or PREMARIN Vaginal Cream (a cream of estrogens)?

- *Estrogens increase the chances of getting cancer of the uterus.*
  Report any unusual vaginal bleeding right away while you are using these products. Vaginal bleeding after menopause may be a warning sign of cancer of the uterus (womb). Your health care provider should check any unusual vaginal bleeding to find out the cause.
- *Do not use estrogens with or without progestins to prevent heart disease, heart attacks, strokes, or dementia.*

- *Using estrogens with or without progestins may increase your chances of getting heart attacks, strokes, breast cancer, and blood clots. Using estrogens, with or without progestins, may increase your risk of dementia, based on a study of women age 65 years or older. You and your health care provider should talk regularly about whether you still need treatment with estrogens.*

In the wake of this first cancer scare, Premarin sales declined. Still, Wyeth-Ayerst was not about to walk away from a billion-dollar market opportunity. The company acknowledged that "unopposed estrogen" could have a carcinogenic effect but countered that the cancer risk could be eliminated if estrogen was balanced with progesterone.

It is true that the progesterone produced by the human body does oppose estrogen and have cancer-protective properties. Unfortunately, pharmaceutical lingo once again confused physicians and consumers by using the terms "progesterone" and "progestin" interchangeably. Progestin is a synthetic version of human progesterone. Later medical studies would show that synthetic estrogen combined with synthetic progestin (trademarked as Provera) was no safer, and possibly even more dangerous, than synthetic estrogen alone.

The Horror Revealed

In 1993, the National Institutes of Health (NIH) initiated a drug trial known as the Women's Health Initiative (WHI). The overall objective of this study was to explore the effects of synthetic combination estrogen-progestin hormone replacement on the long-term health of menopausal women. It involved 16,608 healthy women between the ages of fifty and seventy-nine with an intact uterus (none of these women had had a hysterectomy prior to entering the study). An important objective for the trial was to examine the effect of synthetic estrogen plus progestin on the prevention of heart disease and hip fractures, and any associated change in risk for breast and colon cancer. The study was not designed to address the short-term risks and benefits of hormones for the treatment of menopausal symptoms.

Participants were enrolled in the study between 1993 and 1998 at more than forty clinical sites across the country. Women enrolled in the study were randomly assigned to a daily dose of estrogen plus progestin (0.625 mg of conjugated equine estrogens plus 2.5 mg of medroxyprogesterone acetate), also known by the brand name Prempro. Half the women were given Prempro, while the rest received a sugar pill placebo. Wyeth-Ayerst donated the Prempro.

In 2000 and 2001, WHI investigators complied with a recommendation from the study's Data and Safety Monitoring Board (DSMB) to inform participants of a small increase in heart attacks, strokes, and blood clots in women taking the synthetic hormones. The DSMB, an independent advisory committee charged with reviewing results and ensuring participant safety, found that the actual number of women having any one of these events did not cross the statistical boundary established to ensure participant safety. Therefore, in both 2000 and 2001, the group recommended continuing the trial as they felt that the balance of risks and benefits was still uncertain.

Almost simultaneously, a separate government scientific advisory panel was formed and charged with analyzing the link between synthetic hormone replacement drugs and cancer. In 2001, this panel of experts published an opinion that dramatically contrasted with the DSMB's decision to continue the WHI study. Representatives from the National Cancer Institute and the NIH voted 8-1 to add synthetic estrogen to the nation's list of cancer-causing agents.

Not long after, at the DSMB's regularly scheduled meeting on May 31, 2002, the data from the WHI study revealed that the number of invasive breast cancers had crossed the established signal for risk. Consequently, the WHI study was abruptly halted in July 2002, three years earlier than intended. The initial findings showed that women taking Prempro had an increased risk of heart disease, breast cancer, stroke, and blood clots. The study projected that, for every ten thousand women on Prempro, there would be seven more coronary heart disease events, eight more breast cancers, and eight more strokes than for the ten thousand women taking a placebo or nothing at all. Note that between 30 and 35 percent of the women originally enrolled in the study dropped out due to fear or side effects. Consequently, the number of women projected to suffer potentially critical side effects is most likely skewed to the low end.

Hormone Replacement Therapy

Disease rates for women on hormone replacement therapy (HRT) of estrogen plus progestin or placebo. Annual cases per 10,000 women.

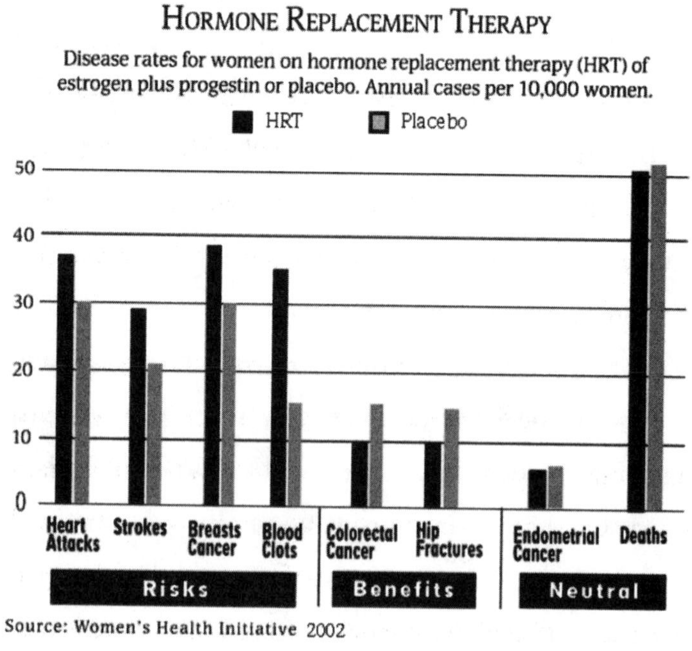

The bad news for synthetic hormone replacement continued. In 2002, the *Journal of the American Medical Association* published another study that was a closer analysis of the WHI findings on the correlation between Prempro and breast cancer. The new research affirmed the breast cancer problem, finding a 26 percent increase in the risk of breast cancer for women taking the synthetic hormone formulation.[5]

In May 2003, additional findings were released indicating that women over sixty-five who were taking Prempro had a heightened risk of dementia or Alzheimer's disease. The WHI also reported that Prempro provided no meaningful improvement in such quality-of-life measures as sleep, emotional health, and sexual satisfaction. The study did find that Prempro provided some relief among women suffering from moderate or severe hot flashes or night sweats.[6]

In addition, the report from the Harbor-UCLA Research and Education Institute found that the cancers tended to be diagnosed at more advanced stages and resulted in substantial increases in the percentage of women with abnormal mammograms. The report of increased risk was not reported with the first findings. Although the breast tumors were most likely already present, they were not detected because synthetic hormones caused increased breast density. In other words, when the women were on Prempro, tumors in their breasts were harder to find. Consequently, when these tumors were detected, the cancer was more advanced.[7]

In the same time frame, a study appeared in the *Journal of the National Cancer Institute* in which Swedish researchers reported that women using synthetic estrogen replacement therapy had a 43 percent increased risk of ovarian cancer. The study went on to report that those women on a combination of synthetic estrogen and progestin had a 54 percent increased risk of ovarian cancer.[8]

Studies published in the last several years continue to be damning. In April 2007, researchers reported that breast cancer rates remained low in 2004 after a substantial decline in 2003. Powerful evidence published in the *New England Journal of Medicine* expressly linked the significant drop in breast cancer rates to the sharp drop in synthetic hormone use by menopausal women. In March 2008, the *Journal of the American Medical Association* published a study which found that women who stopped taking Prempro still had a 24 percent higher risk of developing breast cancer years later.[9]

Big Money at Stake

Media reports about why WHI was so abruptly halted immediately generated panic. With or without their doctor's consent, many women stopped taking synthetic hormones, causing an almost immediate 50 percent drop in sales. Once again on the defensive, Wyeth (formerly Wyeth Ayerst) launched a marketing campaign touting the benefits of a lower dose or different formulation estrogen-progestin therapies. "Go low with Prempro," they chorused. In my opinion, a more honest advertising tag line would read: "Treat your hot flashes and night sweats with *a little less poison.*"

The Battle Is Under Way

To date, more than ten thousand women with breast cancer have sued Wyeth and codefendant Upjohn, a unit of Pfizer Inc. Fifteen cases have been called to trial so far; of those, ten cases have gone to verdict. The other five women received a confidential financial payout in lieu of trial. Eight verdicts have found in favor of the women, two in favor of Wyeth. Pfizer to the date of this writing has not won any verdict in its favor. All verdicts are on appeal. No class-action suits are active at this time. More cases are set for trial in 2009, but the bulk of the cases are not likely to be set for trial until 2010.

2 Bio-Identical Hormone Replacement Therapy (BHRT): A Safe and Effective Alternative

Nannette, a forty-six-year-old single mother of two, walked into my office carrying two women's health books and a file full of Internet research.

I am confused. When my periods became irregular and hot flashes kicked in a little over a year ago, my former gynecologist wanted to put me on Premarin. I had read an article in the newspaper saying it was bad news, so I refused. Instead, I researched natural options on the Internet. I started taking several recommended herbal therapies, but they have done nothing. A friend recommended I read Suzanne Somers's book, The Sexy Years, *and check out what she says about bio-identical hormones. How am I supposed to sort through all this information and find something safe that will work for me?*

Nannette had a right to be confused. In recent years, magazine articles, television shows, and celebrity-written books have bandied around the terms "human," "natural," "herbal," "bio-identical" "BHRT," and "HRT" as if they are interchangeable. They are not. This chapter explains the differences and outlines the medical evidence supporting why bio-identical hormone replacement therapy (BHRT) is the superior choice.

Herbal Remedies Disappoint

According to a 1997 study conducted by the North American Menopause Society, more than 30 percent of women suffering unpleasant menopausal symptoms tried herbal supplements or botanical products such as ginseng, black cohosh, dietary soy, flaxseed, dong quai, evening primrose oil, and wild yam.[1]

Because my patients know that I am a believer in natural medicine, I am frequently asked about these botanical alternatives. I answer with scientific data. While some anecdotal evidence exists that some herbal remedies offer relief for hot flashes and night sweats, there is no strong clinical evidence to support them as a treatment of choice.

Biochemically, these herbal remedies don't work that well for a reason. The body is not set up to convert plant hormones into bio-identical human molecular structures from raw botanical materials. Although natural, the human body cannot recognize and use these herbal remedies.

Bio-Identical Hormones: The Keys That Fit

The hormones that the human body produces travel through the bloodstream to fit into specific hormone receptor sites located throughout the body and brain. Each hormone receptor site recognizes the specific molecular structure of a single type of hormone. A receptor site for progesterone does not recognize estrogen or testosterone, but only recognizes the molecular structure of progesterone.

Human hormones attach to their receptor sites like keys fitting into locks. The chemical term for this key-and-lock phenomenon is relative binding affinity (RBA). Human-produced hormones have a 100 percent RBA for their respective receptor sites.

Bio-identical hormones are derived from precursor molecules of plants (soy or Mexican wild yam) using biochemistry processes in a laboratory. The biochemical process assures that the molecular structure of bio-identical hormones is identical to human hormones. Bio-identical hormones also have a 100 percent RBA for the hormone receptor sites within the body. When introduced into the body, they fit perfectly into the hormone receptor lock and trigger exactly the same response as the one previously fostered by the hormones produced in the ovaries, adrenal gland, or hypothalamus. In other words, at a cellular level the body recognizes, accepts, and uses bio-identical hormones just as it would human hormones.

Synthetic hormones do not have a 100 percent RBA; consequently, they are not keys that fit exactly into the body's hormone receptor locks. At a cellular level, this less-than-perfect fit is the biochemical reason synthetic hormones trigger side effects and sometimes lethal health risks. I quote from the esteemed physician Christiane Northrup in *The Wisdom of Menopause:*

> *Synthetic hormones are made by altering the molecular structure of a hormone enough so that it can be patented. These maintain some of the activity of the natural hormone, but any change in the three-dimensional structure of a hormone, no matter how small, changes its biological effects on the cell in ways that are not completely understood. Frankly, I trust the wisdom coming from Mother Nature's millions of years of experimentation much more than I trust fifty years of bio-chemical wizardry from Father Pharmaceutical!*[2]

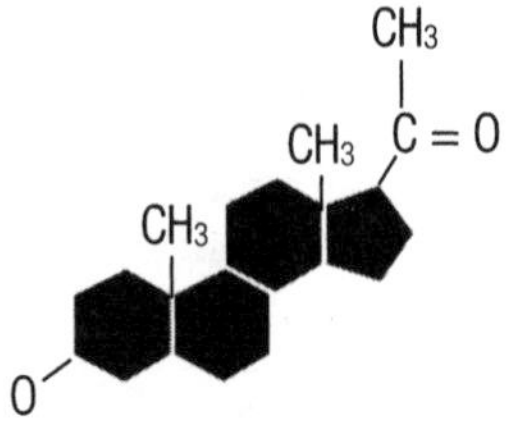

progesterone

Relative Binding Affinity = 100

Source: Human Pharmecology. Third Edition, (1998). Mosely.

The human body possesses progesterone receptors throughout almost all body tissues

The progesterone produced by a woman's ovaries fits perfectly into its receptor as nature intended and elicits the appropriate response.

In pregnancy, the corpus luteum secretes progesterone to support the maturation of the fetus for about ten to twelve weeks, or until the placenta is large enough to take over.

If a pregnancy is at risk during the first trimester, bio-identical progesterone is prescribed to help the body to continue to support the fetus and bring the pregnancy to term.

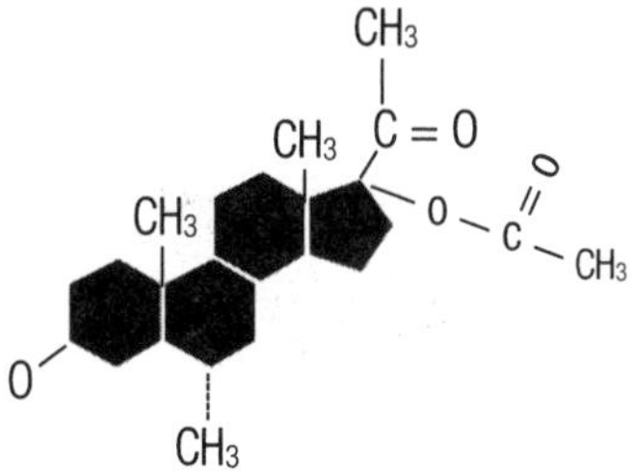

progestin
(medroxyprogesterone acetate)

Relative Binding Affinity = 78

Source: C. W. Randolph, Jr. M.D., R.Ph. May 2006.

The human body does not possess receptors for progestins (synthetic progestrone).

Progestin's RBA is only 78 percent, meaning that this synthetic molecule key does not fit perfectly into the body's hormone receptor locks.

Biochemically, when progestin is introduced into the human system, it confuses the body's cells and receptor sites and stimulates a negative and defensive immune response.

Whereas bio-identical progesterone supports pregnancy, if progestin was administered to a pregnant woman, the pregnancy would be compromised and—if the fetus survived—it would have a significantly higher risk for fetal abnormalities (birth defects).

One Size Does *Not* Fit All

Synthetic hormone drugs are prescribed as if one size fits all. If you are being treated for symptoms of hormone imbalance, you will received the same dosage of synthetic hormone in the same pill whether you are a forty-three-year-old woman weighing 112 pounds or a fifty-nine-year-old woman weighing 225. This approach is dead wrong and dangerous.

A physician prescribing BHRT recognizes that each individual has a unique hormone profile, so one size cannot fit all. For instance, a thirty-five-year-old premenopausal woman has very different hormone-level deficiencies than her fifty-four-year-old postmenopausal neighbor. Consequently, each woman requires a different mix and ratio of BHRT to reestablish her optimum hormonal equilibrium. (Note: The differences between the options for testing hormone levels are discussed in chapter 8.)

Unlike synthetic HRT, an individual's personalized formulation of BHRT is not mass manufactured. Each prescription is compounded on site at a compounding pharmacy. Today's compounding pharmacies can produce literally whatever the doctor orders. Not only do they formulate different dosage strengths—for example, the number of milligrams per gram—they can also incorporate (or mix) the bio-identical hormones into various delivery forms such as capsules, tablets, sublingual drops, gels, or creams.

Compounding pharmacies are different and more specialized than the average drugstore chain on the corner. If you have never heard of a compounding pharmacy before, you should know that every compounding pharmacy is licensed and inspected by the state pharmacy board, and that all materials used in compounded formulations are subject to FDA inspection and the agency's Good Manufacturing Procedure Code.

BHRT: Myths vs. Facts

In an effort to undermine the swelling competition, the pharmaceutical industry has aggressively communicated misinformation about BHRT. The terminology is technical, so it can be difficult for a layperson to sort through and understand. For clarification, I am including the following excerpt of a recent International Academy of Compounding Pharmacies (IACP) rebuttal to three of the common myths that the pharmaceutical promulgates versus BHRT facts:

Myth #1: *The term "bio-identical" is misleading, and "There is no credible science to back the claim that compounded hormones are biologically identical to the hormones produced by the body."*

Fact #1: *Various professional medical societies define the term "bio-identical" as indicating that the chemical structure of a hormone drug is identical to that of the hormone produced by the human body. In the cases of the estrogens estradiol, estrone, and estriol, as well as progesterone and testosterone, the term "bio-identical" accurately characterizes their chemical structure. They are identical to the hormones found in the female and male bodies.*

Myth #2: *No bio-identical hormone replacement therapy (BHRT) product has met federal standards for approval.*

Fact #2: *Since 1986, the FDA has approved at least twelve hormone replacement medications that are bio-identical and marketed as such. Examples of bio-identical hormone drugs manufactured by a select number of forward-thinking pharmaceutical companies include Prometrium, a manufactured progesterone drug approved by the FDA in 1998 and marketed as bio-identical, and EstroGel, an estradiol product approved by the FDA in 2004, which is promoted as "an FDA-approved, bio-identical estrogen replacement therapy."*

Myth #3: *BHRT is unregulated.*

Fact #3: *Bio-identical hormones are made from FDA and the United States Pharmacopeia (USP)–registered materials—the same used by the pharmaceutical manufacturers—and their preparation is well regulated by state boards of pharmacy that have responsibility for overseeing all pharmacy practices in each state.*[3]

Groundbreaking Medical Research

Two years ago I was asked to present on BHRT to a forum on integrative medicine at University of Florida's Shands Jacksonville Medical Center. For weeks prior, my wife and colleague, Genie, and I received threatening phone calls and letters from community physicians incensed that this topic was on a scientific medical meeting agenda. On the day of the presentation, one faculty physician cornered me as I was going on stage. "I will take you down today, you quack," he told me.

Saddened but undaunted, over the next hour I presented current scientific evidence supporting BHRT as the superior treatment of choice for menopausal symptoms as well as symptoms of hormone imbalance presenting at an earlier age. I also offered each physician-attendee a compact disc containing abstracts of more than four hundred medical research studies.

At the end of my talk, I took dozens of questions, including stringent ones from my previously mentioned outspoken adversary. Then my time was up. As I turned to gather my papers, a strange and wonderful thing happened: the auditorium erupted in applause. My eyes welled with tears.

The response of those physicians present was not my victory; it was the victory of medical science over pharmaceutical marketing hype. Eyes were opened, and as a result some physicians would change their habit of routinely prescribing synthetic hormone therapies. Quite possibly, the ripple effect of that day has saved lives.

Why Haven't I (or My Doctor) Heard of Bio-identical Hormones?

If this is the first time you have heard or read anything about bio-identical hormones, you are not alone. In fact, in 2003 the University of California, San Francisco's Women's Health Clinical Research Center released a study reporting that about a quarter of the women who in 2002 stopped taking synthetic hormones when they learned of their risks wound up resuming the dangerous drug regimen because they were miserable and didn't know they had other options.

Greed and ignorance are the primary reasons that you, and possibly your physician, have not heard of bio-identical hormones. From a business perspective, there has been no financial incentive for the pharmaceutical industry to fund medical education forums or launch a national public awareness campaign. Because the Pharmaceutical Research and Manufacturers of America (Big PhRMA) controls much of the funding of large double-blind clinical studies in the United States, a great deal of the research on bio-identical hormones has been done in Europe.

What physician in today's managed-care environment has the time to constantly scour international medical research journals to glean this information? Without adequate education, how is the traditional medical community ever going to change its habit of prescribing synthetic hormone therapies? I challenge our government health agencies, such as the NIH, to secure the funding, foster more studies, and get the word out.

A Crescendo of Informed Voices

The good news is that, since the 2002 output of WHI, the media has done a great deal to raise consumer awareness of BHRT. In 2003, popular women's magazines like

O: *The Oprah Magazine, Good Housekeeping, More,* and *Self* published articles warning of the dangers of synthetic hormone replacement and encouraging readers to challenge their physicians regarding their choices.

Also in 2003, Dr. Phil and his wife, Robin McGraw, broadcast a national TV show titled *Hormones from Hell.* During this program, they interviewed women and a select group of medical experts to discuss the symptoms of hormone imbalance as well as several more natural alternatives to synthetic HRT, including bio-identical hormone therapy. Robin McGraw shared her personal testimony of positive outcomes with BHRT. The show was so enthusiastically received that a sequel was broadcast a few months later.

More recently, actress Suzanne Somers has authored three bestselling books, *The Sexy Years* (2004), *Ageless* (2006), and *Breakthrough* (2008), touting the benefits of bio-identical hormone therapies. These books are based on Ms. Somers's personal experience, as well as the work of physicians and medical researchers across the globe, including my own. While I disagree with the medical protocol Ms. Somers ultimately endorses in *Ageless*, I applaud her willingness to use her celebrity status and mass appeal to ignite a revolt against the entrenched medical establishment's continued prescribing of synthetic hormones.

Many physicians might guffaw to think that their patients would trust medical information gleaned from a celebrity, the Internet, or a TV talk show more than they would their own doctor. No doctor today should be so arrogant or naive. A 2005 study titled National Trends in Healthcare Consumerism found that women make 80.2 percent of their healthcare decisions based on information obtained outside the medical system. Preferred sources included the Internet, media, and word-of-mouth.

While the storm of controversy around hormone replacement continues to rage, I am encouraged by the medical research continuing to prove that BHRT is the superior choice. Even more, I am excited about everyday women who are holding their doctors—and the pharmaceutical industry—to a higher standard. Women across this nation are doing research, banding together, and raising their voices. They are challenging the pharmaceutical industry's control, from their doctors' offices to state courthouses across the United States to the halls of Congress.

Who can oppose the pharmaceutical industry's vast marketing machines with their nearly limitless financial influence on medical research, legislation, education, and prescription patterns?

You can.

PART 2

You Are Not Old, You Are Out of Balance

My hope is you now feel encouraged that with BHRT you have an option for safe and effective hormone replacement. But remember that a critical premise of bio-identical hormone replacement is that each person has a unique hormone profile based on one's individual shifts in hormone production. Your hormone profile will be different from your best friend's or neighbor's. Your personal hormone profile is the sum impact of multiple variables. Chapter 3 describes how age impacts hormone production in women and men. Chapter 4 provides an explanation of how lifestyle issues—such as stress, body fat, sleep patterns, and exposure to environmental toxins—can sabotage hormone balance at any age. A quick and simple hormone Imbalance self-assessment is included. Finally, Chapter 5 looks beyond uncomfortable symptoms to establish the medical link between hormone deficiencies, chronic disease, and decreased longevity.

3 Hormones and Female Life Cycles

Say "hormones" and most people immediately think of either the raging hormones associated with puberty or the waning hormones associated with menopause. The truth is, for women and men, hormones begin their influence on health and quality of life at conception and continue until death. When hormones levels are in optimum ratio, you feel great inside and out. Conversely, when hormone levels are out of balance, you typically feel lousy, you age more rapidly and your health becomes at risk.

YOUR BODY'S HORMONE FACTORY

While our culture is seemingly obsessed with a woman's sexual organs, little awareness is given to the anatomy, physiology, and biochemistry of a woman's body. I remember watching the movie *Fried Green Tomatoes* and chuckling wholeheartedly during the scene when Evelyn Couch, the story's narrator played by Kathy Bates, attended a support group where each woman was challenged to embrace her sexuality by looking at her vagina in a mirror. She was first somewhat horrified, then more than a little fascinated. I felt like Evelyn could easily have been one of my patients who comes into my office and, embarrassed, asks me questions about what was really going on "down there."

Unfortunately, as little as most women know about "down there," they know even less about what is happening "in there"—that is, in the interior of their bodies. Most women who come into my office don't have a clue regarding where their hormones are produced, how they are distributed, or what they do to promote health at a cellular level. To understand the importance of hormone balance, you have to first take a look inside.

The endocrine system is composed of several glands that serve as the body's operational center for regulating hormone production and distribution. If any gland within the endocrine system is not functioning properly, hormone balance is challenged and the whole body suffers.

Your Endocrine Glands at a Glance

To begin to understand the complexity of hormone interactions, it is important to understand the unique function of each gland, its role in hormone production, as well as its interdependent relationship within the endocrine system. In brief:

- *The human body makes hormones from nutrients with the help of enzymes. Cholesterol is the single building-block molecule from which all hormones are derived.*
- *The pituitary and hypothalamus glands are pivotal in regulating the flow of all hormones throughout the body, including estrogen, progesterone, and testosterone. The hypothalamus also directly interacts with the neurotransmitters that regulate mood.*

- *The hypothalamus produces GnRH (gonadotropin-releasing hormone). The pituitary gland produces FSH (follicle-stimulating hormone) and LH (luteinizing hormone). These hormones serve to stimulate the rise of estrogen and progesterone during the monthly menstrual cycle.*
- *The thyroid gland produces the thyroid hormones TSH, T3, T4, and thyroid peroxidase. These hormones are best known for their metabolic function affecting weight.*
- *The two thumb-sized adrenal glands play a critical role in producing hormones and regulating the sympathetic nervous system. One cardinal sign of adrenal exhaustion is relentless, debilitating fatigue. Adrenal glands secrete three hormones in response to stress:*
  1. *Epinepherine, or adrenaline, is the fight-or-flight hormone produced when you think you are being threatened or are in danger.*

2. *Cortisol increases appetite and energy level while taming the allergic and inflammatory responses of the immune system.*
3. *Dehydroepiandrosterone, or DHEA, is often referred to as the anti-aging hormone. It can help protect or increase bone density, keep bad cholesterol levels under control, provide a general sense of vitality and energy, aid natural sleep patterns, and improve mental acuity.*

Sex Hormones in a Healthy Ménage à Trois

Estrogen, progesterone, and testosterone are called the sex hormones. They are primarily produced by the ovaries and testes, but the adrenal glands produce lesser amounts of these hormones. Each sex hormone plays an essential role. When the ratio of each is optimum, or balanced, the three function in a healthy ménage à trios.

In this ideal scenario, estrogen functions to:

- Develop female sex organs and secondary sex characteristics such as breasts and pubic hair
- Maintain the menstrual cycle
- Support the growth and function of the uterus, specifically creating the blood-rich lining of the uterus, preparing it for pregnancy
- Moisturize the vagina and cervix
- Stimulate cell growth

The word "estrogen" is really shorthand for a group of several different but related hormones that perform similar functions within the body. In healthy women who are still menstruating, the amount of each type of estrogen usually fluctuates within the proportions below:

- Estrone/E1 (approximately 3–5 percent of circulating estrogen)
- Estradiol/E2 (approximately 10–20 percent of circulating estrogen)
- Estriol/E3 (approximately 60–80 percent of circulating estrogen)

Progesterone works within the body to:

- Maintain the uterus and prepare it for pregnancy
- Promote survival of the ovum (egg) once fertilized
- Stimulate bone building that can prevent or treat osteoporosis
- Act as a natural diuretic to prevent bloating
- Serve as a natural antidepressant
- Foster a calming effect on the body
- Maintain libido
- Promote regular sleep patterns
- Oppose estrogen's predisposition to promote cell growth so as to provide protection against uterine, breast, and ovarian cancer as well as fibrocystic disease

Although testosterone is often thought of as a male hormone, it actually has several very vital functions within the female body. Testosterone helps to:

- Boost sex drive
- Support feelings of arousal

- Promote a sense of well-being
- Promote muscle strength and healthy body composition
- Increase energy levels
- Increase body hair production
- Produce enlargement of the penis and testes, as well as the clitoris
- Improve bone density

Menstruation and Ovulation

The pituitary gland produces FSH (follicle-stimulating hormone) and LH (luteinizing hormone), and the hypothalamus produces GnRH (gonadotropin-releasing hormone). FSH, LH, and GnRH work together to stimulate the rise of estrogen and progesterone during the monthly menstrual cycle. Estrogen rises in the first half of the cycle, peaks at ovulation, then rises again in the second half along with progesterone. Progesterone is released by the rupturing egg follicle during ovulation. If the egg is not fertilized, then there is no pregnancy and the cycle begins again.

Within the ovaries are the follicles that store a woman's eggs, or ovum. Every month, FSH stimulates the follicles to ovulate. In her early twenties, a woman has approximately four hundred thousand follicles within her ovaries. This high volume of follicles is directly linked to an increased chance of fertilization of the egg, or pregnancy.

By the time a woman enters her thirties, the number of follicles within her body has fallen from four hundred thousand to approximately thirty thousand. While conception is still possible for her, fewer follicles mean fewer eggs, so the odds become increasingly stacked against pregnancy. Physiologically, the reduced quantity of follicles is the reason that many women past their reproductive years require fertility treatment to conceive.

The Aging Ovary

As you age, your ovaries gradually lose their ability to produce the optimum amount of each sex hormone. The shift in balance between the sex hormones occurs in a stair-step fashion. Each descending step is defined by characteristic physical, mental, and emotional symptoms. I call these stair steps "life cycles."

The age range assigned to each life cycle is not absolute. For instance, a forty-five-year-old woman who has not had a period for sixteen months would be menopausal. Similarly, a woman in her early fifties who has irregular periods but whose ovaries still produce enough estrogen for her to ovulate and conceive would be perimenopausal.

The Reproductive Years (the Late Teens Through the Early Thirties)

Physiologically, the late teens through the early thirties are the years when the sex hormones—estrogen, progesterone, and testosterone—are in optimum balance. This age range is called the "reproductive years" because these are the years when ideal levels of all three sex hormones plus an internal repository of over 400,000 follicles (or healthy eggs) prime the female body for conception. At a cellular level, balanced hormone levels mean that women in this age group are also more likely to have high energy and a strong sex drive. A cellular predisposition to want and have the energy for more sex is characteristic of the reproductive years.

Premenopause (Mid-Thirties to Early Forties)

Most women (and their doctors) are unaware that hormone balance issues start in their thirties. As a result, their symptoms are often misdiagnosed and mistreated. Consider Erica, a thirty-seven-year-old working mother of three:

> *Dr. Randolph, my periods are regular, but over the last year and a half, I experienced much heavier bleeding and much worse PMS. I have gained sixteen pounds, I have no sex drive, and I cry all the time. My previous doctor put me on an antidepressant, but it didn't help me feel better. It just made me gain more weight. If I don't get myself together, I am afraid I will sabotage a good marriage. I'm not going through "the Change," but could something else be going on with my hormones?*

Erica's intuition was right. Something was most definitely going on with her hormones.

A woman in her mid-thirties through her early forties who is still regularly menstruating is said to be premenopausal. During these years, the balance of hormones produced by a woman's endocrine system first begins to shift. Progesterone declines and drops 120 times more rapidly than estrogen.

Stable or sometimes increasing estrogen levels combined with decreased progesterone levels create a hormonal disequilibrium or imbalance. The medical term for relatively high estrogen levels and low progesterone levels is estrogen dominance. From their mid-thirties on, almost all women are estrogen dominant.

For the premenopausal woman, common symptoms of estrogen dominance include worsened PMS, breast swelling, weight gain, foggy thinking, mood swings or depression, irregular periods, fluid retention, uterine fibroids, fibrocystic disease, reduced libido, and migraine headaches. Although less common for this life cycle, some women also report hot flashes, night sweats and insomnia.

A shift in the hormones produced by the adrenal glands also begins to shift in the premenopausal years. DHEA levels that peaked in the twenties begin to slowly and steadily decline, dropping 10 percent every decade. Some medical studies correlate the decline in DHEA production with many of the degenerative changes seen in women and men such as heart disease, cancer, and osteoporosis.

Perimenopause (Mid- to Late Forties)

Perimenopause literally means "around menopause." This transition phase can last anywhere from two to eight years; however, women in this life cycle are typically in their mid- to late forties. During perimenopause, progesterone production declines even more significantly while estrogen levels become sporadic, with sometimes very high peaks. Ovaries are still producing eggs although ovulation may be occurring irregularly. Conception is still possible. These are the years when an occasional couple who has grown children in college suddenly discovers that they are going to have an "uh-oh" baby.

Testosterone levels also begin to decline in a woman's forties. A less than optimum ratio of testosterone can result in decreased sex drive, energy level, muscle tone, and vaginal wall thickness. When the vaginal wall is thin, the vagina is less able to lubricate and intercourse often becomes painful.

Menopause (Late Forties to Early Fifties)

A woman is not officially menopausal until she has not had a period for at least twelve months. The average age of women entering natural menopause in the United States is fifty-one years old. Menopause, or "the Change," marks the end of the reproductive years. The pituitary gland and the hypothalamus continue to produce their hormones (GnRH, FSH, and LH), but the ovaries are no longer able to produce enough estrogen to ovulate.

An uninformed medical community continues to regard menopause as an age-related disease, like high blood pressure or Alzheimer's. Another erroneous perception is that menopause is all about estrogen, or lack of it. Even worse is the misconception that, when a woman goes through menopause, her ovaries turn off like a light switch.

The truth is that menopause is not a disease but a natural transition from one life cycle to another. The shift in hormone production that occurs with menopause involves all the sex hormones, not just estrogen. What's more, the ovaries of a menopausal woman are often still quite actively producing between 40 to 60 percent of the estrogen and testosterone produced by a premenopausal woman.

Even though a menopausal woman's ovaries are producing less and less estrogen, the fall of progesterone levels is proportionately much greater. Also, the adrenal glands and body fat continue to produce some estrogen, thereby perpetuating a condition of estrogen dominance. New symptoms of estrogen dominance common to this life cycle include vaginal dryness, hot flashes, hair loss, and night sweats, as well as worsened depression, mood swings, and skin changes.

Hysterectomy and Artificial Menopause

Approximately one in every four American women will enter an abrupt, artificial menopause. The condition known as surgical menopause is the result of a complete hysterectomy. A hysterectomy is the option that most physicians commonly recommend for women who have fibroid tumors, severe endometriosis, cancer, or constant, heavy bleeding. A complete hysterectomy involves surgical removal of the entire reproductive tract, including the uterus, tubes, and ovaries. Unfortunately, up to 90 percent of the time, a woman's pelvic organs will be removed for benign disease that could have been treated by nonsurgical approaches.

Once a woman has had a complete hysterectomy, her body immediately enters menopause regardless of her biological age. Unlike natural menopause, however, after a complete hysterectomy, no ovaries remain to produce any level of hormones. As a result, the body goes into sudden shock.

Too many physicians make the common mistake of prescribing only estrogen for women after a complete hysterectomy, but estrogen alone is not enough. In fact, estrogen triggers estrogen dominance. After a complete hysterectomy, a woman's body needs a new and balanced supply of all her sex hormones: estrogen, progesterone, and testosterone, as well as DHEA.

The thought that the ovaries' production of hormones is not affected by a partial hysterectomy (e.g., removal of the uterus only) is another common error in medical thinking. The ovaries are significantly impacted by a partial hysterectomy because there are two primary pathways for blood flow to the ovaries: one is through the aorta and the second is through the uterus. When the uterus is removed, the flow of blood to the ovaries lessens, and consequently, the production of hormones is reduced. While the hormone imbalance may not be as great as with a complete hysterectomy, women who have a partial hysterectomy should be tested and treated to ensure optimal hormone balance.

Artificial menopause can also occur as a result of radiation or chemotherapy, or by the administration of certain drugs that catalyze menopause for medical reasons (such as to shrink fibroid tumors). Because there is no opportunity for gradual adjustment to the hormonal drop-off, the symptoms of artificial menopause can be sudden, severe, and debilitating, requiring a more immediate intervention of supplemental hormone therapy.

Postmenopause

At fifty-six years old, Betty came to my office as a new patient. "Dr. Randolph," she said, "I went through menopause four years ago but some of my symptoms have never gone away. I still have trouble sleeping, have gained even more weight, and would rather mow the yard than have sex. I have also noticed that now my breasts feel more lumpy and my hair is getting thinner. I thought that once menopause was over, I would be done with all this hormone stuff. What is going on?"

Postmenopausal women continue to have hormone health issues because there are still some hormones circulating within their bodies. Since there is no longer any ovulation, progesterone production drops to almost zero. The ovaries aren't making significant amounts of estrogen, but as with the menopausal woman, the adrenal glands continue to produce some estrogen, though in a lesser amount than previous years. Fat cells also continue to produce some estrogen. Consequently, postmenopausal women are frequently estrogen dominant. Common symptoms of estrogen dominance in this life cycle include a higher risk for breast or uterine cancer, hair loss, postmenopausal weight gain, wrinkly skin, urinary incontinence, low sex drive, cardiovascular disease, and osteoporosis.

After menopause, the ovaries begin to shrink in size, although they never disappear. In some cases, the ovaries of a postmenopausal woman continue to produce a significant amount of testosterone. In fact, the production of testosterone can continue long after the ovaries have significantly decreased their production of both progesterone and estrogen. Is there such a thing as testosterone dominance? Absolutely. Have you ever encountered an older woman with more than a little facial hair and a particularly gruff or deep-sounding voice? Odds are that her ratio of testosterone was much more than optimal.

What About You?

The following table provides a synopsis of hormone issues associated with each lifecycle. Which one best describes you?

Age Range	Life Cycle	Hormone Level Shifts	Medical Condition	Common Symptoms
20s–early 30s	Reproductive years	All hormones at optimum levels	Prime for pregnancy	High libido, high energy, optimum weight and body fat distribution
Mid-30s–early 40s	Premenopause	↓ Progesterone	Estrogen dominance	Worsened PMS, abdominal weight gain, decreased libido, foggy thinking, fatigue, mood swings, depression, headaches, bloating, fibrocystic breasts

Age Range	Life Cycle	Hormone Level Shifts	Medical Condition	Common Symptoms
Mid-late 40s	Perimenopause	↓ Progesterone ↓ Testosterone Estrogen levels high or erratic ↓ DHEA	Estrogen dominant Testosterone deficient	All of the above plus irregular bleeding, hot flashes, night sweats, sleep disturbances, osteoporosis
Late 40s to early 50s	Menopause	↓ Progesterone ↓ Testosterone ↓ Estrogen ↓ DHEA	Deficient in all three sex hormones, but because body is still producing 40–60 percent estrogen, still estrogen dominant	Cessation of menstruation plus all of the above
Mid-50s and beyond	Postmenopause	0 Progesterone ↓ Estrogen but some estrogen produced by adrenal glands and fat cells ↓ Testosterone and DHEA, but ovaries still producing some	Estrogen dominant Possibly also testosterone dominant	All of the above plus increased risk of breast and uterine cancers, fibroids, osteoporosis
Any age	Partial or complete hysterectomy	–0 Progesterone ↓ Testosterone (adrenals continue to produce some) ↓ Estrogen, but some estrogen still produced by fat cells and the adrenals ↓ DHEA	Surgical menopause Estrogen dominant	All of the above

4 The Truth About Male Menopause

While most men think that hormone problems are a woman's thing, the fact is that men also experience a midlife decline in hormone production. Consider the case of Jake, who came to see me at the insistence of his wife, Patti.

Jake started, "I guess Patti told you that I just don't want to 'do it' anymore. I love Patti; she has been my wife and best friend for more than thirty years. And she is still very attractive; tennis and aerobics keep her in great shape. It's just that, at fifty-four years old, I would rather sit on the couch and watch television than have sex."

I asked Jake about his energy level at work. "I have always been regarded as the rising star in the executive team, and my work has even been recognized nationally," he told me, "but, over the last several months, I have started to nod off in important meetings and have little enthusiasm for new projects."

I then asked Jake about his physical activity. While he used to play a couple of rounds of golf or tennis on the weekend and also coach his daughter's soccer team, he reported that he had given it all up. "I am just too tired," he admitted. "I think I am just getting older, but Patti thinks I am depressed. What do you think?"

I believed that Jake's depression, lack of energy, and low libido were all symptoms of an underlying hormonal issue. He was suffering from male menopause, or andropause.

What Is Andropause?

Unlike women, men do not have periods (or lack thereof) as a clear-cut signpost that their hormone levels have shifted. Andropause emerges more subtly. Typically, for a man in his forties, production of testosterone, DHEA, and progesterone begin to decline. Symptoms of male hormone imbalance almost always include low libido and some degree of erectile dysfunction. Other symptoms of andropause are weight gain, lethargy or extreme fatigue, urinary problems, decreased physical agility, and depression.

Andropause is not a new condition. It was first described in the medical literature in the 1940s. Until recently, however, it was not a topic of conversation for either male patients or their physicians. Two factors have helped increase awareness that men go through their own version of the change.

Demographics is the first contributing factor. The number of men over the age of forty-five is close to 40 million today, with the number increasing daily. These baby-boomer males have the mind-set of living a long, productive, and enjoyable life. They have no patience when, during what they regard as the prime time of life, they begin to experience a loss of energy, mental acuity, physical strength, or sexual stamina. Suddenly, these male consumers are asking questions and demanding that the medical community come up with answers.

Viagra, the top-selling prescription drug for erectile dysfunction (E.D.), grossed $521 million in 2003. Television commercials featuring such well-known men as Bob Dole and Mike Ditka endorsing Viagra and Levitra have helped to make E.D. a household term. Men who previously might have cowered with embarrassment now openly compare notes on treatments for erectile dysfunction with their buddies on the golf course.

The women in their lives are also speaking up. Every week at least a dozen or more female patients initiate a conversation with me about their husbands' or lovers' changes in libido, sexual performance, overall energy, or mood. They are relieved to learn that a decrease in hormone production could be the culprit.

The Role of Androgens

Androgens are the male hormones, specifically testosterone and dehydroepiandrosterone (DHEA), that help provide the virility, stamina, and drive most often associated with the male species. They increase energy, decrease fatigue, and help maintain erectile function and normal sex drive. In their anabolic, or building, capacity, they are instrumental in increasing the strength of all the structural tissues—skin, bones, muscles, and heart. A proper balance of the androgen hormones also helps prevent depression and mental fatigue.

Testosterone: The Lead Player

Testosterone is the principal male hormone. It is the primary androgenic hormone and is responsible for the normal growth and development of male sex organs. Testosterone stimulates development of the male secondary characteristics after puberty, including growth of the beard and pubic hair, development of the penis, voice changes, muscle development and contouring of the male body, sex drive, and maturation of the sperm. Finally, testosterone functions to accelerate muscle buildup, increase the formation of red blood cells, speed up regeneration, and help reduce the recovery time needed after injuries.

Testosterone is produced by the Leydig cells in the male testes. Using cholesterol as a base, the testes produce between 4 and 10 mg of testosterone per day. During puberty, testosterone levels are at their lifetime peak. The loss of testosterone, which can begin in a man's thirties, is gradual, with testosterone levels dropping 1 to 2 percent annually. This decline is the result of several concurrent changes. First is a decline in testosterone production consistent with a decline in the number of Leydig (testosterone-producing) cells in the testes as well as decreasing activity of the enzymes that produce testosterone. There is also a diminished response to pituitary signals that normally initiate testosterone production and diminished coordination of the release of the pituitary signals that are produced, decreasing any chance for the testes to continue a normal pattern of testosterone secretion.

Finally, sex-hormone-binding globulin (SHBG) levels increase with age. These proteins cling to testosterone, so even though testosterone may be present, it is not free or biologically available to do its work. Increasing SHBG levels, therefore, reduce free testosterone to a greater extent than the reduction seen in total testosterone. Thus, less total testosterone production in conjunction with increasing binding protein levels act in tandem to synergistically depress free or functional testosterone levels. Unlike the precipitous decline in progesterone levels that women in their thirties experience, the gradual decline in testicular hormone production may take years to exact its mark on a man's physical, mental, and emotional well-being.

For younger men, infertility is often a first sign of post-pubertal testosterone deficiency. The sperm does not mature because the body is not producing enough testosterone. As a man ages, however, the clinical symptoms and signs may evolve slowly and subtly, making them more difficult to detect. Too often, men in their forties or fifties will simply assume that they are "no longer a spring chicken" and just write off the physical, emotional, and mental symptoms of testosterone deficiency. This is not only a sad consequence for a man's quality of life, but if a testosterone deficiency remains undiagnosed and untreated, it can have other longer-term and more severe health effects.

DHEA

DHEA is sometimes referred to as the anti-aging hormone. It is produced in the adrenal glands in men and women, but because DHEA is also produced in the testes, male DHEA levels are about one-third higher. Like testosterone, DHEA levels predictably decline with age. Medical studies have linked abnormally low levels of DHEA with a heightened risk for a number of diseases, including cancer, diabetes, coronary artery disease, obesity, and Alzheimer's. Conversely, supplemental DHEA has been reported in study after study to have a positive effect on the immune system, and to be involved in the prevention of diabetes, cancer, hypertension and obesity.

DHEA was first discovered in 1934. In the early 1980s, DHEA was widely sold in health food stores, primarily as a weight-loss product. Until 1986, DHEA was a nonprescription drug, then the FDA reclassified it on the basis that the longer-term risks were unknown. In October 1994, the U.S. Dietary Supplement Health and Education Act, along with many other events, changed the regulatory status of DHEA so that supplements could again be sold without a prescription.

In the United States, the value of a drug or therapeutic agent is determined by large-scale, double-blind, placebo-based clinical studies, which are very expensive. Like the sex hormones, DHEA is a naturally occurring substance, so its molecular structure cannot be patented. Therefore, pharmaceutical companies have no incentive to invest millions of dollars on clinical trials to determine the effectiveness of DHEA in the treatment of specific diseases, in compliance with the requirements of the FDA for any drug. However, numerous researchers have conducted a wide range of relatively small-scale DHEA studies for many years, and the findings show great promise for the value of DHEA. Interestingly, pharmaceutical firms are reportedly testing synthetic forms of DHEA for their potential in treating AIDS, lupus erythematosus, and Alzheimer's.

The controversy about how DHEA replacement might negatively affect the prostate also plagues many men and their physicians. I address this controversy and others in Chapter 9.

Estrogen Dominance in Men

A man can also be estrogen dominant. I have seen forty-five-year-old men in my practice who are more estrogen dominant than women their age. As men age, their estrogen levels (particularly the form of estrogen called estradiol) gradually rise, and their progesterone and testosterone levels gradually fall. Estrogen dominance occurs because a man's testosterone and progesterone levels are not sufficient to balance the amount of estrogen circulating within his system. In men, estrogen dominance stimulates breast cell growth and prostate hypertrophy—that is, a nontumorous enlargement. Left unchecked, estrogen dominance can cause serious health concerns, such as increased risk of cardiovascular disease, bone density loss, a rise in cholesterol, and urinary and prostate disease.

Are You Andropausal?

Age Range	Life Cycle	Hormone Production	Diagnosis	Symptoms
Men, 40s, 50s, and beyond	Andropause	↓ Testosterone ↓ Progesterone ↓ DHEA	Testosterone deficient Progesterone deficient DHEA deficient Estrogen dominant	Decreased libido and energy, erectile dysfunction, loss of motivation, weight gain, decreased muscle mass, depression, and increased risk of prostate cancer

5 It's Not Just Your Age . . . It's Your Life

The aging body's decreased ability to manufacture optimum amounts of the three sex hormones is a primary cause of hormone imbalance, but you must be aware of other subtle culprits. For instance, consider the case of Paula, a thirty-six-year-old working mother of two:

> *Since I got promoted fourteen months ago, I have been constantly irritable. With my job, two teenagers to watch over, and a house to run, I feel*

as if I am being stalked by a never-ending to-do list. I have also gained thirty pounds because I constantly crave comfort foods, and no matter how much or how often I eat, I never feel full. I have absolutely no interest in sex. In fact, I am hardly ever even in bed. I sleep four or five hours and then work on my computer the rest of the night. No wonder my husband keeps threatening to have an affair.

At thirty-six, Paula's progesterone levels had begun to decline. Still, her symptoms were more extreme than those experienced by most premenopausal women. Something other than age was compromising her hormone balance. From what she had told me, I could guess that stress, body fat, and sleeplessness were her silent saboteurs.

Stress Is a Double Whammy

As you learned in chapter 1, adrenaline and cortisol are two hormones produced by the thumb-sized adrenal glands. These hormones regulate the sympathetic nervous system, influencing mood, energy, sleep, and mental functioning. The amount of each hormone the adrenal glands produce directly corresponds to the amount of stress you experience.

Chronic stress—stress that lasts for more than three months—can upset hormone balance at any age. Modern examples of chronic stress include daily time-management issues, juggling work and family, being laid off or downsized, financial troubles, losing a parent, divorce, angry teenagers, difficult infants, or aging parents. When a young woman like Paula comes to see me complaining of weight gain, low libido, energy loss, sleep disturbances, or are worsened PMS symptoms, I immediately suspect chronic stress as the culprit. For women or men already experiencing symptoms of estrogen dominance, stress-induced hormone imbalance is a double-whammy.

How does stress impact hormone levels? When the brain perceives some form of danger (such as a toddler reaching for a hot pan on the stove or seeing a car suddenly cross over the median and head into your lane of traffic), it signals the adrenal glands to pump out more of the hormone adrenaline, often referred to as the fight-or-flight hormone. The sudden surge in adrenaline levels signals fat cells to quickly release energy. This energy rush stimulates flight, or running away. The adrenaline rush resolves with the passing of the stressful event.

Instead of pumping out more adrenaline, chronic stress causes the adrenal glands to secrete more of the cortisol. Initially cortisol levels are elevated, but if chronic stress is ongoing, the adrenal glands become so exhausted that they are unable to produce even normal amounts of cortisol. When cortisol levels remain too high or too low for an extended period of time, the disequilibrium wreaks havoc on the body. Out-of-normal-range cortisol levels destroy healthy muscle and bone, slow down healing and normal cell regeneration, co-opt biochemicals needed to make other vital hormones, impair digestion, cause abdominal weight gain, dull mental processes, interfere with healthy endocrine function, and weaken your immune system.

The Fat Vise

Body fat is bad for hormone balance. First, when estrogen and progesterone are not properly balanced, you are predisposed at a cellular level to gain weight, particularly around the waist, hips, buttocks, and thighs. Then fat cells produce even more estrogen, thereby worsening your preexisting condition of estrogen dominance. Simultaneously, estrogen dominance causes an increase in thyroid-binding globulin, resulting in a condition of hypothyroidism. Because a primary function of the thyroid is to run the body's metabolism, hypothyroidism causes your body's metabolism to slow down. The result: more weight gain and a vicious cycle of ever-increasing estrogen dominance.

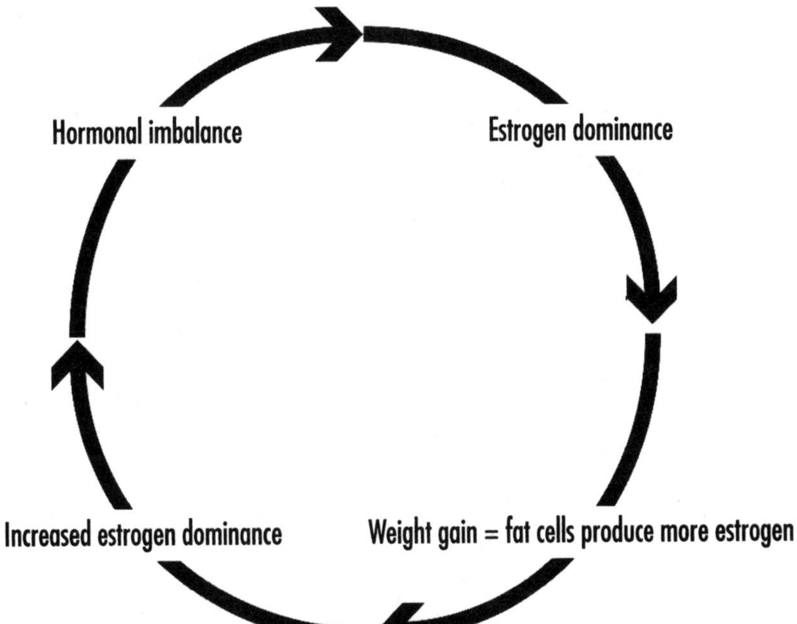

The Domino Effect of Not Enough Sleep

Estrogen dominance frequently causes sleep disorders. Substantial medical evidence suggests a domino effect between estrogen dominance, lack of sleep, and the production of two other hormones: ghrelin and leptin.

According to Michael Breus, a faculty member of the Atlanta School of Sleep Medicine and director of the Sleep Disorders Centers of Southeastern Lung Care in Atlanta, "When you don't get enough sleep, it drives leptin levels down, which means you don't feel as satisfied after you eat. Lack of sleep also causes ghrelin levels to rise, which means your appetite is stimulated, so you want more food."

Living in the United States

Nate, thirty-seven and newly remarried, sat wallowing in despair in my office.

> *I recently married the woman of my dreams, but I have a problem. Nancy is thirty-three years old and this is her first marriage. She wants chil-*

dren, and because she feels her biological clock is ticking, she scheduled physicals for us to ensure that we were both safe to go. Unfortunately, the semen analysis test determined that I have an unusually low sperm count, and now my hormone profile indicates that my testosterone levels are characteristic of a man twice my age. I am still young. What's going on?

Before responding, I asked Nate a few questions about his environment and lifestyle.

Nate worked curing wood chemically in a lumber yard. He kept a plastic bottle of water hooked on his work belt. Most days he brought in leftovers for lunch, covering them in plastic and microwaving before eating. I noticed that Nate's hair was unusually black compared to his salt-and-pepper mustache. When I commented on it, he admitted, "After my divorce, I started dying my hair with one of those drugstore kits for men. I didn't want to look too old to date younger women."

I had the data I needed. Nate's hormone balance and sperm count issues resulted from exposure to environmental hormones.

Xenoestrogens

"Xeno" literally means foreign; therefore, xenoestrogens means foreign estrogens. Xenoestrogens can be found in certain pesticides, herbicides, plastics, fuels, car exhausts, and drugs. Many general hygiene consumer products—such as creams, lotions, soaps, shampoos, perfumes, hair spray, and room deodorizers—contain petrochemicals. These compounds often have chemical structures similar to estrogen and can act like estrogen when introduced into the body. Similarly, industrial solvents are another source of xenoestrogens. Industrial solvents are commonly found in cosmetics, fingernail polish, fingernail polish remover, glues, paint, varnishes, cleaning products, carpet, fiberboard, and other processed woods. Over time, these substances can increase the estrogen load in the body.

Xenoestrogens can be also found in many meats and dairy products because of the form of chemicals and growth hormones given to animals before they are processed for food. In the United States, most ranches inject their cattle and sheep with synthetic steroid growth-promoting hormones. Hormone-treated meat is a very real health issue. More than a decade ago, Roy

Hertz, then director of endocrinology at the National Cancer Institute and a leading authority on hormonal cancers, warned of the carcinogenic risks of estrogenic additives, which can cause imbalances and increases in natural hormone levels.

Phthalates

Phthalates (pronounced thal-ates) are chemicals that soften plastic. That new toy and new shower curtain smell is the smell of phthalates off-gassing. They're also found in medical supplies such as IV tubes and drip bags, plastic food wrapping and containers, and most ubiquitously in fragrances of every description, from scented candles and (so-called) air fresheners, to fabric softeners, perfumes, and nail polish. The highest exposure probably comes from the soft plastics our food is wrapped in (such as the pizza in your freezer) or the plastic water bottles containing our "healthy" water. These plastics leach phthalates directly into the food and drink. The National Resources Defense Council measured phthalates in a variety of air fresheners and found that 80 percent of them contained phthalates.

According to an EPA study published in *Toxicology and Industrial Health*, when female rats were exposed to phthalates, their offspring showed a wide variety of abnormalities. Most striking were their effects as androgen (male hormone) blockers in male offspring, which included a reduction in testosterone levels, abnormalities in the male reproductive tract, and testicular tumors among adult animals. Women exposed to high levels of phthalates have a higher risk of miscarriage.[1]

In adult men, high phthalate levels can cause sluggish sperm and low testosterone levels. Phthalates have also been found to interfere with normal genital development in boys. In the 2003 *Journal of Pediatrics*, an article titled "Pediatric Exposure and Potential Toxicity of Phthalate Plasticizers" noted, "The most sensitive [to the effects of phthalates] system is the immature male reproductive tract."[2] Other medical research studies link common phthalates in our environment with allergies and eczema in children, and early puberty in girls. Most of Europe has already wisely phased out phthalates.

Synthetic Hormone Replacement Drugs and Birth Control Pills

Synthetic hormone replacement drugs, such as the commonly prescribed Premarin and Prempro, and birth control pills both contribute to the development or worsening of estrogen dominance. Many doctors continue to routinely prescribe synthetic hormone replacement therapy for menopausal symptoms such as hot flashes, night sweats, insomnia, and moodiness. These prescription drugs comprise synthetic estrogen or a synthetic estrogen and synthetic progesterone (chemically termed progestin) combination. Synthetic hormone replacement has also been prescribed to protect against the loss of bone after menopause.

Birth control pills also contain synthetic estrogen and progestin. Depending on dosage, they can be very potent, and linger for a long period of time in the body. Birth control pills work by keeping estrogen at such a falsely high level that the body is fooled into responding as if it were pregnant. Therefore, ovulation does not occur.

When the birth control pill (the Pill) was first introduced in 1960, American women and their physicians were quick to embrace it as the contraceptive mode of choice. Within two years, approximately 1.2 million women were using it; within five years, 5 million; and by 1973, about 10 million. In the early 1980s, following reports of possible side effects, use of the Pill dropped to 8.4 million women. Today, however, with low-dose versions available that are purportedly safer, usage is back up and the Pill continues to be the most popular method of nonsurgical contraception. As an FDA advisory committee noted in the mid-1960s, never before or since would so many women take a prescribed drug over such a long period for a reason other than the treatment of a chronic disease.

Fears about blood clots, heart attack, and stroke, which spurred exhaustive research on oral contraceptives in the 1960s and 1970s, have for the most part been laid to rest by the safer, low-dose birth control pills on the market today. Current research suggests that healthy, nonsmoking women have little if any greater risk of these serious health problems than do women who do not use the Pill. Questions about the Pill's association with cancer, however, remain. Some widely reported recent studies support the hypothesis that, in certain groups of women, the risk of breast cancer increases with oral contraceptive use. For instance, one study of more than one hundred thousand women suggests that the increased breast cancer risk associated with birth control pills is highest among women over age forty-five. The study found that the risk of breast cancer was greatest among women age forty-five and over who were still using the Pill. This group of women was nearly one-and-a-half times as likely to get breast cancer as women who had never used the Pill.

In my medical practice today, my nurse practitioners and I counsel patients regarding their options for birth control. For women wanting to postpone pregnancy, we discuss alternatives such as intrauterine devices (IUD) or the Billings ovulation method—a natural method that women can use to monitor fertility based on sensation in the vulva and the appearance and consistency of vaginal mucus discharge. For women who do not want to conceive in the future, we educate about other options, such as a tubal ligation, the Essure method (in which small plugs are inserted into the opening of the Fallopian tubes), or vasectomy for their male partner. For those patients who remain adamant that the Pill is their choice, we continue to prescribe low-dose birth control pills up to age thirty-five for women who are nonsmokers. After age thirty-five, we do not prescribe the Pill because of the previously mentioned studies linking it to an increased risk of breast cancer.

Hormonal Pollutants

Just drinking water out of a faucet may expose you to environmental estrogens and raise your body's internal estrogen levels. According to Marcelle Pick, an obstetrics and gynecology nurse practitioner:

> *Researchers worldwide have observed that fish in our lakes and rivers are actually switching gender due to the high levels of effluent estrogens. Even though mainstream media has only begun to recognize this as "news," experts have been discussing the problem of pharmaceutical pollution for more than twenty-five years, and have known about "gender-bent" fish for more than ten years now! Some surmise these changes to be caused in part by excessive levels of steroids—largely excreted by humans using birth control pills and synthetic*

hormonal replacement therapy. Our water treatment facilities are not designed to remove hormonal pollutants.[3]

As they swim deep beneath Seattle's Elliott Bay, male English sole carry something in their bodies that's not supposed to be there: a protein usually found only in female fish with developing eggs.

These so-called feminized fish, first found in the late 1990s, are thought to be victims of human hormones and hormone-mimicking chemicals—flushed into the water from sewage-treatment plants, factories, storm-water drains, and runoff from roads—that had made their reproductive systems go haywire.

Now a King County study has found that those chemicals, which come from sources as varied as birth-control pills and plastic bottles, detergent and makeup, are more widespread in the region's water than previously known.[4]

Phytoestrogens

Phytoestrogens ("phyto" meaning "plant") are naturally occurring estrogenic compounds that are found in a variety of herbs and spices, such as red clover, black cohosh, chasteberry, and dong quai. Some of the strongest phytoestrogen-containing foods are soy products. These include soybeans, soy milk, tofu, tempeh, textured vegetable protein, roasted soybeans, soy granules, miso, and edamames. Their chemical structure resembles estrogen, but they are much less powerful than human estrogen; their effectiveness represents about one-one thousandth that of the human estrogen produced by the ovary.

Even though phytoestrogens are generally weak estrogens, if you are already estrogen dominant, eating too many phytoestrogens can compound your hormone imbalance problem. Also, phytoestrogenic foods have been found to act as potent antithyroid agents, causing or worsening hypothyroidism.

Quick and Simple Hormone Imbalance Self-Assessment

To determine if you might be the victim of an undiagnosed condition of hormone imbalance, answer the following five questions:

Question #1: How Old Are You?

If you are a woman more than thirty years of age or a man more than forty years of age, your hormone production has begun to shift. If you check two or more of the following symptoms of hormone imbalance and if your symptoms have persisted for more than three months, it is highly likely that your body is signaling that you are suffering from an underlying hormonal imbalance.

Question #2: Are You Suffering from Symptoms of Hormonal Imbalance?

Look at the symptom checklist that follows. If two or more of these symptoms apply to you, and if they have been present for more than three months, it is very likely that your hormone levels are out of balance.

Women

- ☐ Mood swings
- ☐ Hot flashes
- ☐ Night sweats
- ☐ Fatigue
- ☐ Headaches
- ☐ Depressed
- ☐ Anxious
- ☐ Nervous
- ☐ Irritable
- ☐ Tearful
- ☐ Memory lapse
- ☐ Weight gain
- ☐ Premature aging
- ☐ Vaginal dryness
- ☐ Heavy menses
- ☐ Bleeding changes
- ☐ Incontinence
- ☐ Fibrocystic breast
- ☐ Decreased sex drive
- ☐ Tender breast
- ☐ Osteoporosis
- ☐ Water retention

Men

- ☐ Burned-out feeling
- ☐ Abdominal fat
- ☐ Prostate problems
- ☐ Decreased mental clarity
- ☐ Decreased sex drive
- ☐ Increased urinary urge
- ☐ Decreased strength
- ☐ Decreased stamina
- ☐ Difficulty sleeping
- ☐ Decrease urine flow
- ☐ Irritable
- ☐ Depression
- ☐ Erectile dysfunction
- ☐ Hot flashes
- ☐ Night sweats
- ☐ Poor concentration

Question #3: Have You Been Ten or More Pounds Overweight for More Than a Year?

If you have been ten or more pounds overweight for more than a year, your extra body fat is contributing to an underlying condition of hormone imbalance, because fatty tissues within the body make and store estrogen.

Question #4: How Stressed Out Are You?

Review the following list of stress-inducing events. Note that each one has been assigned a Life Change Unit (LCU). To quantify your stress level, first circle all the life events that you have experienced within the last twelve months. Next, add up all the corresponding LCUs. Once you have your LCU Total, find your stress level category. Finally, read how your stress level is linked with hormone imbalance.

Life Event	LCU
1. Death of spouse	100
2. Divorce	73
3. Marital separation	65
4. Jail term	63
5. Death of a close family member	63
6. Personal injury or illness	53
7. Marriage	50
8. Being fired from work	47
9. Reconciliation with spouse	45
10. Retirement	45
11. Change in health of family member	44
12. Illness or change in care needs of a parent	40
13. Sexual difficulties	39
14. Addition of family member	39
15. Major business readjustment	39
16. Major change in financial state	38
17. Death of a close friend	37
18. Changing to a different line of work	36
19. Change in frequency of arguments with spouse	35
20. New loan for major purchase over fifteen thousand dollars	31
21. Foreclosure on a mortgage or loan	30
22. Major change in responsibilities at work	29

Adapted from the work of mental health experts Thomas H. Holmes and Richard H. Rahe

Life Event	LCU
23. Children leaving home	29
24. Trouble with difficult teenagers	29
25. Outstanding personal achievement	28
26. Spouse begins or stops work	26
27. Starting or ending school	26
28. Change in living conditions	25
29. Revision of personal habits (dress, manners, associations)	24
30. Trouble with boss	23
31. Change in work hours, conditions	20
32. Change in residence	20
33. Change in school	20
34. Change in recreational activities	19
35. Change in church activities	19
36. Change in social activities	18
37. Mortgage or loan under fifteen thousand dollars	17
38. Change in sleeping habits	16
39. Change in number of family gatherings	15
40. Change in eating habits	15
41. Vacation	13
42. Christmas	12
43. Minor violation of the law	11
LCU Total Score:	______

Adapted from the work of mental health experts Thomas H. Holmes and Richard H. Rahe

Here is what your LCU Total Score tells you:

If your total is 0–150: At the moment, your stress level is low. The chance of your stress triggering a hormone imbalance is also low.

If your total is 150-300: You have borderline high stress. Your risk for a stress-related hormone imbalance is moderate.

If your total is more than 300: Warning: You have a high stress level. Your chance of having a stress-related hormone imbalance is great.

Question #5: Is Your Environment Putting You at Risk?

If you are living in the United States or Western Europe, your answer should be "yes."

If you have anything in common with the majority of adult American women and men, you just learned that, yes, you are most likely suffering from an underlying hormonal imbalance. Don't despair. You can safely and naturally restore youthful hormone levels and begin to feel like your best self again. Part 3 of this book addresses how to do so, but first I address how hormonal imbalance can affect your health and mortality.

6 More Than Uncomfortable: How Hormone Imbalance Impacts Health and Mortality

At fifty-six years old, Sandra officially entered menopause. "I haven't had a period for sixteen months now, and I can tell you one thing for sure: menopause isn't for sissies. I feel worse than ever. I never sleep through the night, have several overwhelming hot flashes a day, feel bloated even when I pee every ten minutes, and would rather change my cat's litter box than have sex. Still, I am not one of those women who whine and go to bed. I'm going to be tough and literally sweat this out. It's not like I am sick or anything."

Like Sandra, many women and men believe that, while their symptoms of hormone imbalance might be irritating, they have no real health consequence. This thinking is dangerous. The medical reality is that, over the long term, conditions of estrogen dominance and testosterone deficiency have been directly linked to an increased risk of several chronic diseases, including cancer, cardiac disease, stroke, and Alzheimer's. Even more potent: an untreated hormone imbalance has the potential to shorten your life span.

Estrogen Dominance Increases Risk of Chronic Disease

An overabundance of estrogen circulating within the body can be deadly. As previously described, one of estrogen's functions within the body is to foster cell proliferation or growth. Progesterone, on the other hand, inhibits cell growth. When progesterone levels begin to decline and the body becomes estrogen dominant, cell growth continues unchecked.

Estrogen Dominance and Female Cancers

The close relationship between the risk of cancer and exposure to estrogen continues to be reviewed and validated. Multiple studies show that women who develop breast cancer tend to have higher estrogen levels than women without breast cancer. Other studies have documented that women who had been treated for breast cancer who continued to have high estrogen levels had a return of the disease sooner than breast cancer survivors with lower estrogen levels.

Another study found that women who start menstruating at an early age, or who enter menopause at a later age, are at greater risk for developing breast cancer. This data supports the theory that the number of menstrual cycles a woman has, and hence the length of exposure to estrogen during her lifetime, is a critical factor impacting breast cancer risk.

Estrogen dominance can lead to cancer in one of two ways. The first has to do with the concentration of each of the three different forms of estrogen—estrone, estradiol, and estriol—circulating within the body. Estrone and estradiol both work within the body to increase expression of a gene (BCL-2) that causes cell division (development and growth), particularly in hormone-sensitive tissue such as the breast or uterine lining. If unchecked, this cell proliferation can lead to cancer. In fact, nearly every risk factor for breast and uterine cancer can be either directly or indirectly linked to an increase in estrone, estradiol, or their receptor activity. A study published in the March 2008 issue of *Cancer Epidemiology, Biomarkers and Prevention* determined that high levels of estradiol were associated with significantly higher incidence of breast cancer recurrence.[1]

Premarin, the synthetic HRT manufactured by Wyeth-Ayerst, is composed of 49.3 percent estrone, almost ten times the ratio that occurs naturally within the body. Is it any wonder that this drug was found to increase risk of invasive breast cancer by 41 percent?

The second factor influencing your cancer risk has to do with how your body metabolizes its estrogen. Very simply, estrogen can be metabolized down a "bad" pathway—one that is more cancer inducing—or a "good" pathway—one that is more cancer protective. The chemical name for the "bad" pathway is 16-hydroxyestrone. On the other hand, 2-hydroxyesterone and 2-hydoxyestradiol are the "good" pathways. Each woman's estrogen metabolism is different, so the balance between your "good" and "bad" estrogen pathways is unique. The balance of anti- and pro-carcinogenic estrogen may be investigated with a urine test (trademarked Estronex). The lower your 2/16 ratio, the greater your cancer risk.

Treating Hormone-Dependent Breast Cancer

If you are diagnosed with breast cancer, a hormone receptors assay can determine if your cancer is sensitive to estrogen or progesterone. A cancer is called "ER-positive" if it has receptors for estrogen. It is called "PR-positive" if it has receptors for progesterone. An ER-positive tumor is more likely to grow in a high-estrogen environment. ER-negative tumors are usually not affected by the levels of estrogen in your body. Breast cancers that are either ER-positive or PR-positive, or both, tend to respond well to hormone therapy.

ER-positive cancers are more likely to respond to anti-estrogen therapies. Commonly prescribed regimens include selective estrogen receptor modulators (SERMS), such as Tamoxifen or Evista, that block circulating estrogen from binding with its receptor. Another approach is aromatase inhibitors, such as Arimidex or Femara, that inhibit the conversion of testosterone to estrogen. While these therapies can be effective, they have their downside. SERMS can have an estrogenic effect that can cause cancer of the uterus. Aromatase inhibitors frequently cause debilitating side effects, including bone and joint pain, vaginal atrophy, or osteoporosis. Chrysin and melatonin are two naturally occurring aromatase inhibitors that work without the harsh side effects previously mentioned.

Having treated patients with ER-positive cancers for more than a decade, I always obtain a complete hormone level profile, including current estrogen levels, prior to initiating any form of therapy. I then monitor impact of the chosen anti-estrogen regimen very closely. For patients within five years of their diagnosis, I obtain a follow-up hormone level profile every three months. For patients beyond five years, I obtain follow-up hormone level profiles every four to six months. I know of no oncologist who does the same thing, which I find mind-boggling.

Estrogen Dominance and Prostate Cancer

The late John R. Lee, M.D., commonly regarded as the father of the bio-identical hormone replacement movement, believed estrogen dominance to be the primary cause of prostate enlargement and prostate cancer in men.[2] Current research studies validate that when prostate cells are exposed to estrogen, the cells proliferate and become cancerous. Since the male prostate is the embryonic equivalent of the uterus, these finding should not be surprising.

Estrogen Dominance, Belly Fat, Chronic Disease, and Early Mortality

You've already learned that estrogen dominance causes abdominal weight gain and that fat cells produce even more estrogen. Recent medical studies link this hormone-related middle-age spread to multiple health risks.

According to a March 2008 study in the *Journal of Neurology*, belly fat in your forties can boost your risk of getting Alzheimer's or other dementia decades later.[3] Similarly, output of a study released by the National Institutes of Health (NIH) indicated that women who carry excess fat around their waistlines are at greater risk of dying early from cancer or heart disease than those with smaller waistlines.[4] Finally, a recently released German study found that people with bigger waist circumferences (greater than forty inches for men and thirty-five inches for women) had four times the stroke risk when compared with people with smaller waistlines.[5]

Estrogen Dominance and Your Brain

A variety of evidence suggests a link between estrogen dominance and migraine headaches, anxiety disorders, insomnia, and decreased mental acuity. Recent research has also suggested that an imbalance between estrogen and progesterone levels may be a precursor to Alzheimer's disease.

> *No, you are not losing your mind: you're just losing much-needed progesterone. When you don't have enough progesterone circulating, estrogen is*

the dominant hormone. Estrogen in overabundance makes you angry, edgy, short-tempered, and anxious. At the same time, estrogen increases the water content of the cells in your brain making you groggy, fuzzy, and unfocused.

Erika Schwartz, M.D., in *The Hormone Solution* (2002)

Low Testosterone Levels, Higher Death Risk for Men

As a board-certified gynecologist, I didn't open my practice expecting men to be a large segment of my patient base. Initially, I referred male patients to a urologist or internist, but in follow-up conversations I discovered that their condition of testosterone deficiency would either be ignored or misdiagnosed. Recognizing once again that the traditional medical community's ignorance was putting lives in jeopardy, I opened my doors. Today, one out of every three patients I see is a male.

While testosterone is most frequently associated with sex drive, low testosterone levels are a big red flag for other health issues. Low testosterone levels have been found to be more common in men with heart disease. In one study, men with confirmed heart disease had lower testosterone levels than healthy control subjects. Men with the most severe heart disease had the lowest testosterone levels. Conversely, a number of studies reveal that higher testosterone or DHEA levels are associated with reduced heart attack risk. There is further evidence that low testosterone levels are a risk factor for the later development of metabolic syndrome and diabetes.

When it comes to disease and death, medical ignorance can be cruel. In November 2007, the *American Heart Association* released the following data linking testosterone levels to incidences of disease and death:[6]

Testosterone Blood Levels and Subsequent Incidences of Disease and Death

	Highest testosterone	Next to hightest testosterone	Next to lowest testosterone	Lowest testosterone
All-cause mortality	41% reduction	38% reduction	25% reduction	Highest rate of death
Coronary heart disease	48% reduction	41% reduction	29% reduction	Highest rate of death
Cancer	29% reduction	23% reduction	26% reduction	Highest rate of death

Another landmark study analyzed the relationship of circulating free testosterone, DHEA, and insulin-like growth factor (IGF-1) to death rates in men suffering from chronic heart failure. The results speak for themselves:[7]

Hormone Status	Three-Year Survival Rate
High levels of DHEA, testosterone, and IGF-1	83%
Deficiency in one hormone (testosterone, DHEA, or IGF-1)	74%
Deficiency in two hormones (testosterone, DHEA, or IGF-1)	55%
Deficiency in all three hormones (testosterone, DHEA, or IGF-1)	27%

The Danger of Frequent Misdiagnosis

Genie and I are passionate about our mission to educate consumers and their physicians about hormone health because the stakes are high. When symptoms of hormone imbalance are ignored or treated with a Band-Aid, such as synthetic hormones, antidepressants, or oral medications for erectile problems, health becomes at risk, quality of life can be sabotaged, and longevity is compromised. The good news is that BHRT treats the underlying issue, not just the symptom. Read on to learn how.

PART 3

Three Steps to Feel—and Look—Younger and Better

Are you concerned about putting all this medical science about hormone health into an easy action plan? Don't worry. The encouraging news is that it is medically possible for you to turn back the clock to feel—and look—more like yourself again. Age-related hormone decline can be safely and effectively treated with BHRT, and stress-induced hormone imbalance can be reversed with lifestyle changes.

The next three chapters detail a straightforward three-step plan to balance your hormones and help you get your life back. Chapter 7 describes why progesterone is the most important—and most frequently overlooked—hormone. Chapter 8 establishes the critical premise of BHRT: always replace only the hormones your body is missing. Finally, chapter 9 tells you how to make hormone-healthy choices every day.

7 Step #1: Start with Bio-Identical Progesterone

Carol came to see me for the first time at age forty-four. She complained of irregular and heavy bleeding, hot flashes, night sweats, weight gain, low libido, and foggy thinking.

"I know my hormones are a mess," she told me. "I bet you will have to empty your pharmacy to get me feeling better. Go ahead. I am so desperate that I'll take two of everything on the buffet."

Analysis of Carol's lab work indicated that she was

highly estrogen dominant, but all her other hormones were in normal range. When I told her that she would require only bio-identical progesterone cream to restore her optimum hormone balance, Carol was skeptical.

"That's it?" she queried. "Just a little cream every morning and evening? As bad as I feel, are you sure progesterone cream is all I need?"

I encouraged Carol to give the progesterone cream a try for at least two weeks. If her symptoms persisted after that time, I advised her to come back in so that I could adjust her prescription. Otherwise I would see her in three months for a follow-up consultation.

Three months to the day Carol was back in my office sharing her glowing report.

"My periods are regular again, and the bleeding is back to my normal monthly flow. I can sleep through the night without waking up in a dank sweat and feeling like I need to wring my pajamas out in the sink."

She went on, "I have lost twelve pounds and can fit into my skinny pants again. I'm not edgy and snapping at my family like I was before."

Progesterone Comes Center Stage

For years, estrogen has been the focus of most conversations about hormones. Through his books and speaking, Dr. John Lee was the first to foster a wide-scale awareness of progesterone's critical role. Now, because of breakthrough medical research, progesterone is moving center stage.

What the Research Shows

Exciting new medical studies provide clear physiological and biochemical evidence substantiating how optimum progesterone levels contribute to overall health and well-being. For instance, a prospective, randomized, double-blind, placebo-controlled, crossover study funded in part by the American Heart Association and published in the July/August 2008 *International Journal of Pharmaceutical Compounding* showed that, unlike the synthetic estrogens and synthetic estrogen plus synthetic progestin drugs used in WHI that were linked to an increased risk of cardiac disease and stroke, bio-identical progesterone was shown to relieve menopausal symptoms without compromising cardiac or vascular health.[1]

A sentinel study published in the 2005 issue of the *International Journal of Cancer* showed that use of bio-identical progesterone in hormone therapy regimens did not affect the risk of developing breast cancer, while the use of synthetic progestins increased this risk. In fact the bio-identical progesterone was found to decrease a woman's risk of breast cancer by 10 percent.[2]

In contrast to evidence linking synthetic hormones to an increased risk of Alzheimer's, multiple medical research studies offer groundbreaking evidence that bio-identical progesterone can play an important role in promoting and enhancing repair after traumatic brain injury or stroke.[3]

Other scientifically proven health benefits of bio-identical progesterone are as follows.

Cancer-Protective

Over the past three decades, Dr. Joel T. Hargrove, former chief of the Department of Gynecologic Reproductive Endocrinology at Vanderbilt University Medical Center, has published multiple studies validating the efficacy of bio-identical progesterone replacement in many highly reputed medical journals, including *Obstetrics and Gynecology* and the *International Journal of Gynecological Pathology*. The clinical trials conducted by Dr. Hargrove evidenced the critical role that progesterone plays in suppressing estrogen-dependent cell proliferation that can be a precursor for the development of cancerous tissue. Dr. Hargrove's work provides evidence that when bio-identical progesterone balances estrogen dominance and turns off the cell growth mechanism, it can have a cancer-preventing effect.

Breast Health

Breast cancer is the most frequently diagnosed cancer in women. Many breast cancers are also hormone dependent. As previously described, estrogen increases proliferation of breast cells, and when uncontrolled, this cell proliferation results in cancer. Very simply, continuous exposure to high levels of unopposed estrogens definitely increases a woman's risk of getting breast cancer. The body has "too much estrogen" anytime the body's production of estrogen is not in equilibrium with its production of progesterone.

In contrast, progesterone functions within the body to inhibit cell proliferation. Studies in such highly respected clinical journals as the *Journal of the National Cancer Institute,* the *International Journal of Cancer, Fertility and Sterility,* and the *American Journal of Epidemiology* and Endocrinology have validated the anticarcinogenic properties of progesterone.[4] Today the statistics are that one out of eight women in the United States will be diagnosed with breast cancer. Early detection of breast cancer is very important, but prevention is a much more critical opportunity.

The scientific result I would most like to see would show a reduction in the incidence of breast cancer because every woman in the United States had begun to augment her body's production of progesterone with bio-identical progesterone as soon as her hormone levels began to shift.

Cardiac Health

Progesterone is good for heart health. Because heart disease is the number-one killer of women in America, the effect of progesterone on cardiac health has also been an area of extensive research. Recall that the Women's Health Initiative (WHI) trial indicated synthetic estrogen plus progestin (synthetic progesterone) increased cardiac risk. The good news is that researchers have proven that for women on a hormone replacement regimen that includes both estrogen and bio-identical progesterone, progesterone actually serves to reduce coronary vascular activity. In other words, whether progesterone is produced within the body naturally or is a bio-identical formulation added back into a woman's system, progesterone has definitively been shown to balance estrogen and have a cardio-protective effect. Multiple studies continue to validate the beneficial effect that bio-identical progesterone has on cardiovascular function.[5]

Osteoporosis

Bone density loss (osteoporosis) is another health concern for many women today. Bone tissue breaking down and rebuilding continuously is normal, as it is for all the cells in our bodies. This process takes place when osteoclast cells dissolve old bone tissue (osteoblast cells, on the other hand, stimulate new bone growth). Estrogen has a rate-limiting effect on osteoclasts: it only delays the breakdown of bone tissue. Bio-identical progesterone, on the other hand, stimulates osteoblast cells (bone formation cells) that result in new bone growth.

Morris Noteloviz, M.D., Ph.D., author of *Stand Tall: Every Woman's Guide to Preventing and Treating Osteoporosis*, states, "Progesterone receptors are present in osteoblasts. Based on in vivo [in the body] and clinical studies, it is now believed that progesterone may stimulate new bone formation, although the mechanism has not yet been identified." Women using transdermal [transferred into the bloodstream through the skin] bio-identical progesterone cream experienced an average of 7 to 8 percent bone mineral density increase in the first year, 4 to 5 percent in the second year, and 3 to 4 percent in the third year. Untreated women in this category typically lose 1.5 percent bone mineral density per year. With regard to the treatment and prevention of bone density loss, no other form of HRT or dietary supplementation has had as high a level of positive response as bio-identical progesterone.[6]

PMS

Have you or anyone you know ever suffered from premenstrual syndrome (PMS)? Well, if so, here is news about progesterone that you will want to hear. In the early 1950s, a theory was advanced within medical communities that PMS was caused by unopposed estrogen during the luteal phase of the menstrual cycle (the time between ovulation and the onset of the next menses). To test this theory, researchers administered bio-identical progesterone by intramuscular injection, vaginal or rectal suppository, or subcutaneous pellets. Progesterone resolved PMS symptoms in 83 percent of the women included in the study.[7]

Weight Gain

Estrogen dominance causes weight gain. The weight itself is only part of the problem. Body shape changes because the fat accumulates around the stomach, buttocks, and thighs rather than being more evenly distributed over the entire body. Once again, progesterone can effectively address the biochemical reason for this weight gain.

Too much estrogen also causes tissues around the abdominal area to retain water, or bloat. In younger women, this bloating is most noticeable around their menstrual cycle when their progesterone levels naturally drop to precipitate menstruation. As women age and their progesterone levels do not cycle back up during the month, then the resulting estrogen dominance causes the bloating to be a constant issue. This uncomfortable feeling is eliminated when progesterone balances the estrogen. Progesterone then acts as a natural diuretic, thereby reducing the bloating.

Changes in blood sugar levels that occur with age and as a result of hormone imbalance are also linked to weight gain. As the body's production of progesterone decreases and circulating estrogen becomes dominant, insulin is released more rapidly and more often. When fluctuating hormones unnaturally stimulate insulin release, the body craves sugar. Food cravings can sometimes be uncontrollable. Many women report that they find themselves consuming many more sweets, even when they are not truly hungry. As a result, they ingest more calories than their bodies require. When progesterone is in balance with estrogen, it serves to temper insulin release, thereby normalizing blood sugar levels and reducing food cravings.

Sex Drive

In his groundbreaking book, *What Your Doctor May Not Tell You About Menopause*, Dr. John R. Lee explains that he was intrigued about the underlying biochemical reason that so many women experienced a loss of sex drive with age. Dr. Lee indicates that his anecdotal findings prompted him to further investigation. When his patients took a saliva test, he found that their low libido frequently corresponded with a progesterone deficiency. Over the past decade, several studies have validated Dr. Lee's premise and confirmed a positive correlation between progesterone levels and sexual interest, desire, and response.

Quality of Life

Similar findings of progesterone improving overall quality of life have been reported by other nationally recognized centers of medical excellence. For instance, in the

May 2000 issue of the *Journal of Women's Health*, the Mayo Clinic published a study reporting that women who included naturally occurring (bio-identical) progesterone in their hormone replacement regimen were more satisfied with their overall quality of life. Investigators followed 176 women whose prescribed hormone replacement therapy included bio-identical progesterone with estrogen. They determined that, unlike synthetic progestin, bio-identical progesterone did not negate the positive effect that estrogen can have on cholesterol levels.

Study participants also reported that they felt an improvement in several other health areas as a result of their progesterone therapy. According to Dr. Lorraine Fitzpatrick, a Mayo Clinic endocrinologist and the leading investigator of the study, "We already knew that progesterone can decrease some of the risks of estrogen replacement therapy such as increased risk of endometrial or uterine cancers. Now it seems that naturally-occurring (bio-identical) progesterone can also reduce the occurrence of sleep disorders, hot flashes, anxiety, and symptoms of depression."[8]

When It's Safe to Self-Diagnose and Treat

Like Carol (whom you met at the opening of this chapter), sometimes all you need to eliminate a condition of estrogen dominance is bio-identical progesterone. I have found that 70 to 80 percent of premenopausal women experiencing symptoms of estrogen dominance can safely self-treat their condition with over-the-counter bio-identical progesterone cream.

Bio-identical progesterone is very safe, and side effects are rare. The most common side effect is drowsiness. Bio-identical progesterone creams can be found in most health food stores or over the Internet. The good news is that they are available. The bad news is that you don't always know what you are getting. Most product labels do not specify whether or not they meet the following criteria for product excellence:

- Is the progesterone truly bio-identical?
- Do the hormones used in the formulation meet the United States Pharmacopoeia (USP) gold standards for quality and purity?

- Was the progesterone product actually compounded under the strict guidelines approved by the National Association of Compounding Pharmacists?
- Some topical formulations suspend the bio-identical progesterone in oils that are not easily absorbed into the skin. Is the type of oil in the cream formulation one that will promote or inhibit transdermal absorption?

My Natural Balance Cream meets all the above criteria and is available through our website, www.hormonewell.com. In addition, a listing of other over-the-counter bio-identical progesterone creams I have reviewed and approved for quality and safety is included in the Appendix.

The concentration of bio-identical progesterone in most over-the-counter creams is 15 to 20 milligrams per 1.25 grams of cream. I have found that more consistently favorable results are obtained when a higher concentration of bio-identical progesterone is used. My personal formulation—Dr. Randoph's Natural Balance Cream—contains 25 milligrams of bio-identical progesterone per 1.25 grams of cream, or 1 pump.

Follow package directions when using any over-the-counter product; however, if not noted, always apply any bio-identical progesterone cream above the waist. A recent Australian study showed that transdermal progesterone applied below the waist or on the legs can get into the liver through collateral circulation. This liver pass-through effect decreases effectiveness.

When bio-identical progesterone is applied topically, it is absorbed transdermally (through the skin) immediately into the bloodstream and then distributed and utilized in progesterone target tissues. Transdermal absorption allows the body to receive, recognize, and utilize bio-identical progesterone in exactly the same manner it would the progesterone produced by the body's own ovaries. Biochemically, you couldn't ask for anything better.

Some women find that over-the-counter bio-identical progesterone cream is all they ever need. For others, the over-the-counter formulation works for awhile, then symptoms come back. When symptoms return, it is a signal that the production of other hormone levels has shifted and now the body needs something more. Consider the following:

Dr. Randolph's Natural Progesterone Cream Application Instructions

- Apply cream twice daily, morning and evening to area marked "1" in the figure below. The next day choose another numbered area and apply twice daily to that area.
- Continue rotating site of cream application, moving to another numbered area each day. Repeat rotation of cream application sites.
- **Always use progesterone cream twice daily.** Using progesterone cream alone is safe. CAUTION: If you still have your uterus, do not take estrogen without progesterone. This may cause pre-cancerous cells to form in the uterine lining. REFILL INSTRUCTIONS: Call refills in directly to the dispensary at (904) 694-1271 or email refill requests to: rx@cwrandolph.com. Please leave your name, date of birth, daytime telephone number, prescription number or brief description of what you are requesting.

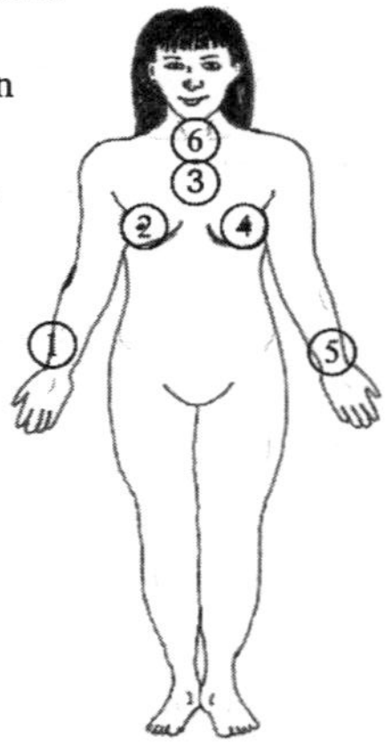

Application Areas:
#1 = Right forearm
#2 = Right breast
#3 = Chest
#4 = Left breast
#5 = Left forearm
#6 = Neck

PMS: Use 1 to 2 pumps twice a day from days 8-26 of your cycle.

Osteoporosis: Use 1 to 2 pumps twice a day for 25 days, and then take 5 days off. Repeat. After 3 months, decrease to 1/2 to 1 pump twice a day. If using with estrogen, use every day of the month.

Endometriosis: Use 2 pumps twice a day from days 6-26 of your cycle.

Ovarian Cysts: Use 1 to 2 pumps twice a day from days 8-26 of your cycle.

Fibrocystic Breast: Use 1 to 2 pumps twice a day from days 8-26 of your cycle.

Uterine Fibroids: Use 1 to 2 pumps twice a day from days 8-26 of your cycle.

Pre or Peri-Menopause: Use 1 to 2 pumps twice a day from days 8-26 of your cycle. If using with estrogen, use every day of the month.

Post-Menopause or Hysterectomy: Use 1 to 2 pumps twice a day for 25 days. Then take 5 days off. Repeat. After 3 months decrease to 1 pump twice a day. If using with estrogen, use every day of the month.

Men: 45 years and older, use 1/8 of teaspoon or 1 pump twice a day.

NOTE: First day of bleeding is the first day of your cycle. If you have additional questions, please visit www.hormonewell.com.

At forty-seven years of age, Pam walked into my consultation room for the first time. She was obviously frustrated. "Dr. Randolph, three years ago I started using your progesterone cream. I couldn't believe the results. In just two weeks I started losing weight, felt calmer, stopped having so many headaches, and began to sleep through the night. Over the last six months, however, it has stopped working. I have gained fifteen pounds, feel constantly edgy, and have begun having hot flashes and night sweats. What's going on? Did you change your progesterone cream formula?"

The formula had not changed, but Pam's hormone balance had. The return of Pam's symptoms was a red flag that she was no longer suffering from only a deficiency in progesterone. As occurs with all women as they age, the production of her other sex hormones had also begun to decline. Now, to treat Pam's underlying hormonal imbalance and eliminate her symptoms, I would require a comprehensive analysis of all her hormone levels. Once I had Pam's personalized hormone level profile in-hand, I could prescribe an individualized formulation of each of the bio-identical hormones she would require to re-establish her body's optimum hormonal equilibrium.

8 Step #2: Get a Personalized Prescription for BHRT

Megan, a forty-nine-year-old mother of three and grandmother of one, cornered me one night in a neighborhood restaurant.

"Dr. Randolph," she said, "you don't know me, but I live next door to Jennifer More, who has been your patient for more than ten years. Jennifer knew my husband and I were having some problems, so she lent me her testosterone drops, hoping they might put me in the mood to do something other than yell at him. My sex drive has improved, but I have also grown a mustache. Jennifer doesn't have one. Why do I?"

Despite her good intentions, Jennifer was wrong to have shared her prescription bio-identical testosterone drops with her friend. Bio-identical hormones are not youth in a cream or sex in a bottle. They are individualized prescriptions whose strength, or concentration, is based on the exact amount of each hormone you will need to bring your hormone levels back into optimum balance.

Jennifer, now fifty-seven, had gone through menopause five years earlier. Her personal hormone profile indicated a deficit of all three sex hormones: estrogen, progesterone, and testosterone. At forty-nine and still regularly menstruating, Megan was perimenopausal. Lab results confirmed that Megan's body was producing adequate amounts of testosterone on its own. By taking Jennifer's testosterone drops, Megan had catapulted her system into a condition of testosterone dominance. The extra testosterone circulating within Megan's system was responsible for her new facial hair growth, but the damage could have been more serious. Hormone levels that are not in the physiologic realm and that are above normal limits can be harmful.

While the concept behind BHRT sounds simple, effectively analyzing hormone levels and prescribing individualized doses of BHRT can be complex.

Your Personal Hormone-Level Profile

A complete and individualized hormone-level profile is needed to provide a rational basis for correcting anything more than the initial downshift in progesterone production. Your hormone-level profile should include measurements of free, or bio-available, and total hormones.

When the endocrine system manufactures sex hormones (estrogen, progesterone, and testosterone), they are released into the bloodstream bound to carrier proteins. Only a small fraction (1 to 5 percent) of a given amount of a sex hormone breaks loose from the carrier protein in the bloodstream and is free to enter the target tissues. This free or unbound hormone is bio-available to act on target tissues such as the breast, uterus, brain, and skin. Bio-available hormone levels can be tested using blood, saliva, or urine.

In addition to determining the bio-available levels of the sex hormones, a complete hormone profile must include analysis of the other hormones not bound to carrier proteins. These include the thyroid hormones (TSH, T3, T4, and thyroid peroxidase) and the adrenal hormones (cortisol and DHEA).

Recently, newer, more ultrasensitive blood tests called radio-immune assays (RIA) give an accurate reading of both bio-available and other required hormone levels, thereby providing a complete hormone level in a single test. In other words, an RIA is a one-time, one-stop-shop, giving you everything you need for a personalized hormone-level profile.

Saliva testing accurately measures tissue levels of the bio-available sex hormones but it cannot measure levels of other important hormones, such as FSH, LH, or the hormones produced by the thyroid gland (TSH, T3, T4, and thyroid peroxidase). To obtain a complete hormone profile, salivary tests must be augmented with a finger-stick dried blood spot test.

A urine sample can provide a complete hormone profile if analyzed with gas chromatography coupled with mass spectrometry (GC/MS). This testing modality is used to detect illicit steroid hormone use among athletes, including those participating in the Olympics. However, owing to high equipment and personnel costs associated with this still rather sophisticated equipment and methodology, this testing modality has largely been confined to universities and medical schools.

Interpreting a hormone profile is not the work of amateurs. You will need the help of a qualified medical professional.

Finding a Doctor

The most frequent question received on our Natural Hormone Institute of America website, www.hormonewell.com, is "How do I find a doctor practicing near me who is knowledgeable about BHRT?"

The good news is that, because of the crescendo of consumer demand, an increasing number of physicians across the country are learning about and prescribing BHRT. Both Genie and I are on the faculty of two national BHRT continuing medical education (CME) programs, one offered by ZRT Labs and one by Professional Compounding Centers of America (PCCA). In 2004, there might have been only 20 to 30 physicians registered for a CME program; the rest of the audience would be compounding pharmacists. Beginning in 2006, attendance swelled to more than 120 physicians. Even better, these doctors are not showing up just for a few hours or a weekend. They are committing to a learning program that can span a year as it moves them through increasing levels of competence.

Here's the bad news: some doctors are getting into BHRT as a marketing strategy. These doctors recognize the demand factor but, instead of attending comprehensive CME programs or committing to a strenuous tutorial with a nationally recognized medical expert, they are going to a three- to four-hour seminar and then calling themselves "BHRT experts." Each week I see patients whose BHRT treatment regimen I have to clean up because their original prescribing physician was not sufficiently knowledgeable about the intricacies of hormone production and physiologic dosing. As a result, the patient's symptoms were not alleviated, but worsened.

Here are three tips for getting help you can trust:

1. *Don't trust your health to amateurs.* Ask your local compounding pharmacist which doctors in your area are skilled in BHRT. If you need help finding a compounding pharmacy in your area, contact one of the two organizations listed below.

   The International Academy of Compounding Pharmacists (IACP)
   P.O. Box 1365
   Sugar Land, TX 77487
   Phone: 281-933-8400
   Fax: 281-495-0602
   Website: http://www.iacprx.org

   or

   Professional Compounding Centers of America (PCCA)
   9901 South Wilcrest Drive
   Houston, TX 77099
   Phone: 877-798-3224
   Fax: 877-765-1422
   Website: http://www.pccarx.com

2. *Look beyond marketing.* Just as I have urged you to not trust pharmaceutical marketing, I encourage you to be skeptical about physician advertising. I do not mean that any physician who advertises can't be trusted; in fact, my Ageless and Wellness Medical Center is frequently featured in local magazines and directories. When it comes to your health, however, I want you to find out more than what you will read in any ad or brochure. Ask the doctor:

    - How long have you been diagnosing and treating patients with symptoms of hormone imbalance with BHRT?
    - Where and with whom did you train? (Do an Internet search of their response and check out the source.)
    - Understanding the legalities of patient privacy, do you have two to three patients who would be comfortable speaking with me regarding their experience?
    - Which compounding pharmacy do you use to fill your prescriptions?

3. *Gather your data.* Keep a diary of your symptoms, copies of all your lab work, and records of any prescription's strength and dosage form, and take notes during and after any consultation.

Available Dosage Forms

As I described in the previous chapter, over-the-counter bio-identical progesterone is available only in a cream base. A stronger concentration of bio-identical progesterone is also available by prescription, which can be formulated into a cream or capsule. Though transdermal absorption is excellent, I frequently recommend taking additional bio-identical progesterone in capsule form at bedtime to control heavy or irregular bleeding. Also, some patients report that they just can't remember to use a cream and prefer an oral dosage form.

Estrogen and testosterone are also best absorbed transdermally, but can be administered in different formulations. These include capsules, gels, creams, lozenges, drops, suppositories, and injections. It should be noted that testosterone is poorly absorbed orally.

For patients requiring supplementation of multiple hormones, I recommend that each hormone be administered in its own formulation. That way, if the patient's response is not optimal, the concentration of the one needing adjustment can be find tuned without disturbing the desired strength of the one(s) that is working. Some physicians and compounding pharmacists prefer to combine all hormones in a single formulation because they feel a single regimen enhances patient convenience and compliance. That is all well and good, but if the original prescription requires adjustment, you have to start over, essentially tossing the baby out with the bathwater.

Physiologic Dosing

Analysis of your personal hormone-level profile determines which bio-identical hormones you need, as well as the optimum dosage for each one. The options include one or more of the estrogens (estriol, estradiol, estrone), progesterone, testosterone, and DHEA. I cannot emphasize strongly enough that *no woman, with or without a uterus or ovaries, should ever take estrogen of any kind alone*. It should always be balanced with bio-identical progesterone.

When I start a patient on a regimen of bio-identical progesterone only, I typically retest hormone levels in three months unless symptoms persist. For patients prescribed more than one bio-identical hormone, I typically retest hormone levels in four to six weeks. If levels have not been elevated to optimum range, or if my patient is still bothered by symptoms, I then adjust her or his BHRT prescription. Once hormone levels are stable and my patient asymptomatic, I recommend testing again in three months and then a recheck once a year unless old symptoms recur or new ones emerge. Symptoms should be regarded as an alarm clock letting you know that hormone balance has once again shifted and something more, or different, is now needed.

Chapter 2 told you that "one size does not fit all" is a central theme of BHRT. In practice this means that one fifty-two-year-old woman might require bio-identical progesterone and bi-est, a combination of estriol and estradiol. Another fifty-two-year-old woman might require bio-identical progesterone plus testosterone. Two women might need supplementation of the same hormones but in different strengths. One man may need only testosterone while the next requires testosterone, progesterone, and DHEA. BHRT prescriptions are compounded on the spot because each prescription is individualized.

Just as one size does not fit all, when it comes to BHRT it is also important to recognize that one size probably won't fit forever. The production of your hormones will continue to decline, causing an ongoing shift in hormone balance. For most women, the mix of BHRT they need during premenopause years will be different than the mix of BHRT needed to restore optimum hormone balance postmenopause. Similarly, most men will need their dosage of testosterone or DHEA adjusted with age.

A Controversial Approach for Women

The Wiley Protocol for bio-identical hormone replacement gained notoriety after being advocated by Suzanne Somers in *Ageless*. The Wiley Protocol was first devised and advocated by T. S. Wiley, author of *Lights Out: Sleep, Sugar, and Survival* and *Sex, Lies, and Menopause*. The protocol claims to relieve the symptoms of menopause but is also promoted as an approach to increasing overall health. It involves using rhythmic doses of hormones to re-create a premenopausal woman's monthly cycle; in other words, it uses high dosages of bio-identical hormones to force a menopausal woman to continue to have periods.

While Ms. Somers interviewed and quoted me in *Ageless*, I did not endorse the Wiley protocol. As I stated earlier, I applaud Ms. Somers for her willingness to use her celebrity status to raise awareness about BHRT, but I have grave concerns about the protocol that she has embraced. The Wiley Protocol uses high, nonphysiologic dosages of hormones that many medical experts agree could be dangerous. Furthermore, Ms. Wiley's lack of any formal medical education or training makes me question her competence in designing a medical protocol. Finally, significant side effects have been reported by women on this protocol.

Bio-Identical Testosterone and Men: Contraindications and Precautions

For men, bio-identical testosterone can be easily administered and monitored as part of a complete proactive health program. Analysis of testosterone levels gives enough clinical information to make a decision as to whether or not replacement of this hormone is indicated; however, some relative contraindications must be kept in mind.

Prostate cancer is an absolute contraindication for testosterone supplementation. Prostate cancer is the leading cancer in men, with about 180,000 new cases diagnosed each year. Patients often have no symptoms and are taken by surprise when a nodule is discovered in an exam or a high prostate-specific antigen (PSA) is revealed in bloodwork.

I always order bloodwork for prostate cancer prior to initiating any bio-identical testosterone therapy. Some tests are more sensitive for identifying patients with cancer and others are more specific, meaning that fewer patients without cancer test false positive. Unfortunately, none of the available tests is perfect. All will miss a percentage of cancers (false negative), and all will incorrectly identify some patients who prove not to have cancer (false positive). I order both the Total and Free PSA.

The Total PSA test, which measures nanograms of PSA per milliliter of blood, is a more sensitive test. The drawback is that the more sensitive the test, the more likely that the result is a false positive. The Free PSA test, which measures the percentage of PSA that is not bound to proteins in the blood, is more specific, which means that fewer patients without cancer test false positive.

A more accurate, next-generation prostate cancer test is a urine-based genetic test for prostate cancer. The PCA3Plus, validated by Bostwick Laboratories Inc., predicts prostate cancer with a sensitivity of 91 percent.

Many men are concerned that testosterone supplementation will impact their prostate. It will not if administered in physiologic doses and monitored appropriately. First and foremost, testosterone alone does not cause prostate enlargement, or benign prostatic hypertrophy (BPH). The danger to the prostate occurs when testosterone is metabolized into two different hormones, estradiol (E2) and dihydrotestosterone (DHT) by two different enzymes:

aromatase and 5-alpha reductase, respectively. For some men, an exaggerated rise in E2 may even produce breast enlargement. This conversion of testosterone to E2 and DHT can be safely blocked with medication.

Seldom-occurring male breast cancer is another contraindication for bio-identical testosterone replacement therapy. Sleep apnea syndrome or obstructive pulmonary diseases may be enhanced by testosterone therapy, so I regard these as relative contraindications to be factored into my decision—as well as my patient's—as to whether it would be prudent to proceed.

If no contraindications are present, the next step is to decide the delivery mode. There are several different options including sublingual (under the tongue), injectable, topical, and implantable formulations. Clinically, I have found the injectable form of bio-identical testosterone to be the delivery mode of choice. An intramuscular injection safely elevates testosterone levels without side effects. The dosage can be easily monitored and managed via follow-up testing of hormone levels. Studies indicate that delivering testosterone this way has a 100 percent success rate in providing usable hormone.

Testosterone pellets have also been developed that can

provide augmented serum testosterone levels for up to six months. These pellets require a very minor in-office surgical procedure for implantation and prove to be a good option for many people. I've been doing hormone pellet insertion for more than twenty years. Low testosterone levels may also be supplemented indirectly by the administration of human chorionic gonadotropin, which stimulates testosterone production by the testes.

Ongoing monitoring of hormone levels is a must. If testosterone levels are kept too high, hemoglobin and hematocrit levels may also indicate a preeminent condition called polycythemia, where the body produces too many blood cells. Testosterone levels that are too high can also upset cholesterol metabolism, potentially exacerbating high blood pressure.

9 Make Hormone-Healthy Choices

BHRT is an essential component of my approach to rebalance your hormones, but it is not a magic potion allowing you to overstress, shortchange a good night's sleep, or eat a never-ending stash of chocolate bars and potato chips without consequence. For optimum health and well-being, you need to augment any BHRT regimen with informed lifestyle choices supporting your hormone health goals. This chapter provides a simple framework you can put into action every day to keep your life—and your hormones—as balanced as possible.

Boost Your Adrenal System

Stress is a common denominator of modern-day living. I do not know of any person who is not challenged by something, whether it is financial worries, a too long to-do list, relationship tensions, or the fear of being suddenly alone. Chapter 5 described how long-term stress exhausts your adrenal system and upsets the balance of other key hormones, most significantly cortisol and DHEA.

The best way to boost your adrenal system and support its optimum hormone production is to stress less and rest more. The concept is basic, but making it work in your life can be daunting. I suggest you experiment with multiple stress management approaches and find one or more that help you feel calmer and more centered. Make this a daily habit, and you will go a long way toward keeping stress from sabotaging your hormone balance.

Exercise

Regular exercise is one of the best physical stress-reduction techniques available. Exercise not only improves your health and reduces stress, it also relaxes tense muscles and helps you to sleep. Exercise has a positive impact on hormone balance and can cause release of chemicals called endorphins into your bloodstream. These give you a feeling of happiness and positively affect your overall sense of well-being.

To avoid boredom, I recommend that each person create their own toy-box approach to exercising. For instance, in a given week you may choose to walk, run, box, swim, dance, work out at the gym, take a Pilates class, play a round of golf, or participate in a tennis match or racquetball game. What matters is that you move, get your heart rate up, and stay motivated.

The Relaxation Response

The Relaxation Response is a technique developed by Herbert Benson, M.D., at Harvard Medical School. It has been tested extensively and is explained in detail in *The Relaxation Response* by Dr. Benson. The technique works. Set aside ten or twenty minutes today and try it. Sit quietly in a comfortable position, then:

1. Close your eyes.
2. Deeply relax all your muscles, beginning at your feet and progressing up to your face. Keep them relaxed.
3. Breathe through your nose. Become aware of your breathing. As you breathe out, say the word "one" silently to yourself. For example, breathe in . . . out—*one*; in . . . out—*one*; in . . . out—*one*, and so on. Breathe easily and naturally.
4. Continue for ten to twenty minutes. You may open your eyes to check the time, but do not use an alarm. When you finish, sit quietly for several minutes, first with your eyes closed and later with your eyes opened. Do not stand up for a few minutes.
5. Do not worry about whether you are successful in achieving a deep level of relaxation. Maintain a passive attitude and permit relaxation to occur at its own pace. When distracting thoughts occur, try to ignore them by not dwelling upon them and return to repeating *one*. With practice, the response should come with little effort.

Practice the technique once or twice daily, but not within two hours after any meal, since the digestive process seem to interfere with the body's ability to fully relax.

Yoga

The practice of yoga involves stretching the body and forming different poses while keeping breathing slow and controlled. The body becomes relaxed and energized at the same time. There are various styles of yoga, some moving through the poses more quickly, almost like an aerobic workout, and other styles relaxing deeply into each pose. Some have a more spiritual angle, while others are used purely as a form of exercise.

Yoga has been widely recognized for its psychological benefits, including stress reduction and a sense of well-being. If you are a novice, I recommend that you first take a class or work one-on-one with an instructor to learn how to move into the poses without injuring yourself. Once you know the basics, yoga poses can be done just about anywhere, and a yoga program can go for hours or minutes, depending on your schedule.

Walking Meditation

Connecting with the vastness of nature has a way of putting daily trials and tribulations in perspective. Genie and I are blessed to live near the ocean, so mindful walks on the beach are a regular part of our stress-management practice, but you don't have to live near the water or mountains to tap into the calmness and comfort that nature can provide. Here's a simple approach to a walking meditation:

1. Find a park or stretch of natural beauty.
2. Wear comfortable walking shoes.
3. Bring water—preferably in a bottle (non-phthalate) that is on a shoulder strap or can be hooked to your waistband, allowing your hands to move freely and rhythmically as you walk.
4. Turn your cell phone off and put in your pocket. Use only for emergencies such as a sprained ankle.
5. Focus on feeling your feet on the ground and the air coming into your lungs. Repeat.
6. Notice other living things—trees, animals, flowers, children—but don't stop to talk. This is time only for you.

7. When your mind starts to bring up issues, actions, or concerns, tell yourself, *Not now. I'll pick that back up later.*
8. Check your energy level when you are done. Most people report feeling more energy and less stress.

Count Your Blessings in Your Car

What if you considered your car to be your personal prayer closet? This is one of Genie's favorite ways to destress and refocus on what is working in her life versus what needs fixing. She recommends the following:

1. Turn off the cell phone and radio.
2. Speak out loud about two or three things in your life for which you are grateful.
3. Repeat, but pause after naming each item to consider how it contributes to feelings of health, well-being, love, joy, comfort, peace, safety, or prosperity.
4. Choose to regard traffic stalls or red lights as a way the Universe is slowing you down.

5. Once at your destination, say a prayer of thankfulness before getting out of the car.

Eat to Eliminate Extra Estrogen

Your diet directly impacts your hormone balance. As you have learned, body fat produces extra estrogen. The good news is that you can choose foods that will function within your body to reduce an unhealthy estrogen load. Even better, they will help you lose those unwanted pounds that all the extra estrogen in your system has caused you to pack on.

Cruciferous Vegetables and Indole-3-Carbinol (I3C)

In chapter 6, you learned that there are good and bad estrogens. How estrogen is metabolized in the body is determined by an individual's biochemical makeup, with some people producing more 2-hydroxy derivatives (the "good" estrogens) and others producing more 4- and 16-hydroxyesterone (the "bad" estrogens). Consuming large amounts of cruciferous vegetables, such as broccoli, asparagus, cauliflower, spinach, Brussels sprouts, celery, beet root, kale, cabbage, parsley root, radish, turnip, and collard and mustard greens, has been shown to improve the production of "good" estrogen and foster an optimum 2/16 estrogen ratio.

Biochemically, here's what happens. Cruciferous vegetables contain a phytonutrient called Indole-3-Carbinol (I3C). I3C has been shown to act as a catalyst to pull estrone down a benign pathway to 2-hydroxy estrone, thus decreasing levels of the carcinogenic 4- and 16-alpha hydroxyestrone. In lay terms, cruciferous vegetables can help decrease the body's load of unhealthy estrogens and reduce an overall unhealthy condition of estrogen dominance.

Citrus Fruits: D-Limomene

D-Limomene, found in the oils of citrus fruits, has been shown to promote detoxification of estrogen. Common citrus fruits include oranges, grapefruit, tangerines, lemons, limes, and tangelos. Research also found that, when administered an extract of D-Limomene, both male and female lab mice evidenced lower body weight.

Insoluble Fiber

There are two types of fiber: soluble and insoluble. Soluble fiber dissolves in water and is degraded by bacteria in your colon. Soluble fiber forms a gel in your intestines that regulates the flow of waste material through your digestive tract. This type of fiber is found in oatmeal, oat bran, dried peas, beans, lentils, apples, pears, strawberries, and blueberries. Soluble fiber is good for you, but no matter how much of it you eat, it won't influence your hormonal equilibrium.

Insoluble fiber, on the other hand, can directly impact your hormone balance by helping decrease estrogen overload. Insoluble fiber binds to extra estrogen in the digestive tract. This extra estrogen is later eliminated in the body through the feces. According to the Harvard School of Public Health, sources of insoluble fiber include whole grains, whole wheat breads, barley, couscous, brown rice, whole-grain breakfast cereals, wheat bran, seeds, carrots, cucumbers, zucchini, celery, and tomatoes.

Lignans

Ground or milled flaxseed, sesame seeds, and flaxseed oil are part of a food group called lignans. The friendly bacteria in our intestines convert plant lignans into the "human" lignans, primarily enterolactone, that have a weak estrogen-like activity. When there are low estrogen levels in the body, these weak lignan "estrogens" make up some of the insufficiency. When the body is estrogen dominant, however, the lignan "estrogens" bind to the human body's estrogen receptors, thereby reducing human estrogen activity at a cellular level.

Eat Organic

Organic foods are better food choices because they are free of synthetic hormones and other chemicals used by mass food producers to force an unnatural growth cycle. Still, many people worry that buying organic adds up at the cash register. Here are some simple tips to help you eat organically and stay within budget:

1. *Understand why organic foods should be an important part of your diet.* Organic foods are

grown with no chemical or hormonal additives in their growth cycle or fewer than in conventionally grown produce and meat. Laws on organic labeling in many places ban the use of a wide array of pesticides, fungicides, herbicides, hormone treatments, antibiotics, and so forth on any produce or meat destined to carry an organic certification.

2. *Choose the crucial dozen organic foods.* The dozen foods listed here are considered to be the foods most vulnerable to the addition of too many pesticides, growth hormones, antibiotics, and so on. For these foods, home washing and cooking practices do not significantly reduce your exposure to chemical or hormonal residues.
   - Beef, chicken, and pork
   - Dairy products: milk, cheese, and butter
   - Strawberries, raspberries, and cherries
   - Apples and pears
   - Tomatoes
   - Spinach and salad greens
   - Coffee
   - Potatoes

- Stone fruits: peaches, nectarines, and apricots
- Grapes
- Celery
- Peppers (capsicums), green and red

3. *Shop around.* Organic foods can be pricey if you just shop in your supermarket, but you probably have more choices for organic food in your community than you realize. All it takes is a little research.

To find a source of organic foods near you or to order online, check out the following websites: www.organicfoods.com, www.organicconsumer.org, www.eatwell.com, and www.diamondorganics.com. Also, local farmers' markets can be a great source for organic foods, often at lower prices than you would pay in the supermarket or health food store.

What About Supplements?

Over the last several years, I have researched and tested scores of nutritional supplements to ascertain their true mechanism for beneficially influencing healthy estrogen metabolism and optimum adrenal gland function. Today I recommend a select group of supplements to enhance healthy hormone balance.

Calcium D-Glucarate

Calcium D- Glucarate is a natural substance that promotes the body's detoxification process and supports hormonal balance. Calcium D-Glucarate facilitates the detoxification process by inhibiting the reabsorption of estrogen-like toxins into the bloodstream, allowing them to leave the body and be excreted in the feces.

Calcium D-Glucarate has been found in animals to lower unhealthy estrogen levels and thereby inhibit the development or progression of cancer. I recommend taking 1000 mg of Calcium D-Glucarate twice daily.

Diindolymethane (DIM)

DIM is a phytonutrient akin to the Indole-3-Carbinol (I3C) found in cruciferous vegetables. DIM has unique hormonal benefits. It supports the activity of enzymes that improve estrogen metabolism by increasing the levels of 2-hydroxyestrone—the "good" estrogen. When taken as part of a healthy diet, I have found that DIM helps support PMS symptoms, fat loss, and healthy estrogen metabolism.

In men, DIM also promotes its own metabolism, allowing for greater testosterone activity. Men taking DIM supplements will benefit biochemically as DIM promotes an optimal testosterone-to-estrogen ratio. I recommend 200 mg of DIM each day.

The B Vitamins

The B vitamins—B1, B2, B3, B5, B6, B12, and folate—do a lot within your body to support estrogen detoxification. Conversely, if your body is deficient in B vitamins, you will have higher levels of circulating estrogens.

B vitamins also impact estrogen activity for the hormone receptors at the cellular level. Clinical studies have shown that high levels of intracellular B6 can decrease the binding response at the estrogen hormone receptor site. What happens at the cellular level is sort of like an internal game of musical chairs: if the music stops and B6 sits down in the "estrogen chair," then the estrogen molecule is out of the game.

Because the B vitamins work together to perform such vital tasks at the cellular level, I recommend that you take the entire B-complex, not just one or two of the vitamins. To treat symptoms of hormone imbalance, you need between 50 and 100 mg of B-Complex that contains 50 mgs of thiamine (B1), riboflavin (B2), niacin (B3), pantothenic acid (B5), B6, PABA, choline, and inositol; 50 mcg of B12; and 400 mcg of folic acid.

Vitamin E

I remembered from my limited nutritional studies in medical school that, years ago, researchers studied the effects of Vitamin E in reducing the effects of menopause and that most studies found Vitamin E to be helpful.

Vitamin E has been shown to reduce PMS-related breast tenderness, nervousness, depression, headache, fatigue, and insomnia. I had a hunch I knew why. As I reviewed the more current medical literature evaluating the health benefits of Vitamin E, I was validated when my hunch proved to be correct.

Low Vitamin E levels were linked to estrogen dominance. Furthermore, Vitamin E deficiency has been found to inhibit estrogen detoxification. I recommend taking 800 IU per day of Vitamin E: 400 IU in the morning and 400 IU at bedtime.

Calcium-Magnesium Combo

Most women and men find it difficult to get 1,200 to 1,500 mg of needed calcium from their diet. As a rule, I recommend supplementing calcium intake with a calcium-magnesium combination supplement.

Magnesium helps the body eliminate excess estrogen. For women, magnesium levels tend to fall at certain times during the menstrual cycle. These shifts in magnesium levels can upset an optimum calcium-magnesium ratio. In proper balance, the body better absorbs and assimilates the calcium it needs and allows calcium to migrate out of tissue and organs where it doesn't belong.

Without magnesium, calcium may be not fully utilized. Underabsorption of calcium can lead to menstrual cramps. Similar to a vitamin E deficiency, when the body does not have enough magnesium to support calcium absorption, many women report PMS symptoms such as mood swings, fatigue, headaches, and sleeplessness.

Premenstrual chocolate craving is a phenomenon that has puzzled a great many physicians. They have been unable to explain why some women have this overwhelming urge to eat lots and lots of chocolate right before their periods, yet at other times of the month their chocolate cravings remain under control. When I started thinking about it, the PMS-chocolate connection made a lot of sense. Chocolate is very high in magnesium.

Keeping an optimal balance of calcium and magnesium is critical for optimal physical functioning and for hormone balance. I recommend that each day you take a calcium-magnesium supplement that combines these minerals in a ratio of two parts calcium (1,500 mg) to one part magnesium (750 mg).

READER/CUSTOMER CARE SURVEY

HEFG

We care about your opinions! Please take a moment to fill out our online Reader Survey at **http://survey.hcibooks.com**.
As a **"THANK YOU"** you will receive a **VALUABLE INSTANT COUPON** towards future book purchases as well as a **SPECIAL GIFT** available only online! Or, you may mail this card back to us.

(PLEASE PRINT IN ALL CAPS)

First Name | MI. | Last Name

Address | City

State | Zip | Email

1. Gender
❒ Female ❒ Male

2. Age
❒ 8 or younger
❒ 9-12 ❒ 13-16
❒ 17-20 ❒ 21-30
❒ 31+

3. Did you receive this book as a gift?
❒ Yes ❒ No

4. Annual Household Income
❒ under $25,000
❒ $25,000 - $34,999
❒ $35,000 - $49,999
❒ $50,000 - $74,999
❒ over $75,000

5. What are the ages of the children living in your house?
❒ 0 - 14 ❒ 15+

6. Marital Status
❒ Single
❒ Married
❒ Divorced
❒ Widowed

7. How did you find out about the book?
(please choose one)
❒ Recommendation
❒ Store Display
❒ Online
❒ Catalog/Mailing
❒ Interview/Review

8. Where do you usually buy books?
(please choose one)
❒ Bookstore
❒ Online
❒ Book Club/Mail Order
❒ Price Club (Sam's Club, Costco's, etc.)
❒ Retail Store (Target, Wal-Mart, etc.)

9. What subject do you enjoy reading about the most?
(please choose one)
❒ Parenting/Family
❒ Relationships
❒ Recovery/Addictions
❒ Health/Nutrition
❒ Christianity
❒ Spirituality/Inspiration
❒ Business Self-help
❒ Women's Issues
❒ Sports

10. What attracts you most to a book?
(please choose one)
❒ Title
❒ Cover Design
❒ Author
❒ Content

TAPE IN MIDDLE; DO NOT STAPLE

NO POSTAGE
NECESSARY
IF MAILED
IN THE
UNITED STATES

BUSINESS REPLY MAIL

FIRST-CLASS MAIL PERMIT NO 45 DEERFIELD BEACH, FL

POSTAGE WILL BE PAID BY ADDRESSEE

Health Communications, Inc.
3201 SW 15th Street
Deerfield Beach FL 33442-9875

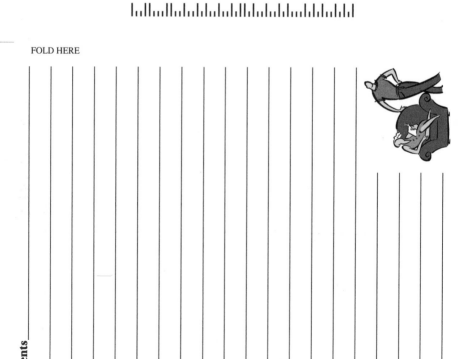

FOLD HERE

Comments

Certain supplements can nourish stress-depleted adrenal glands while encouraging adrenal cortex secretions, which help to maintain optimal hormone balance. I have developed an Adrenal Boost formula, designed to increase overall body energy while decreasing exhaustion and fatigue. It is helpful for people who are under stress because it supports the glands responsible for the discretion of energy flow. The ingredients in my Adrenal Boost formula include vitamin C, vitamin B6, pantothenic acid, deglycyrrhized licorice root, Mexican wild yam root, schizandra berry, Eleutherococcus senticosus root, stinging nettle leaf, trimethylglycine, special plant cellulose, natural silca, vegetable stearate, and magnesium stearate. I recommend taking one capsule every morning and every night. Note: Do not use if you have high blood pressure; this products contains licorice root, which can elevate blood pressure.

7-Keto Dehydroepiandrosterone (DHEA)

Dehydroepiandrosterone (DHEA) is one of the hormones produced by the adrenal glands. Stress and aging can both cause a decline in healthy DHEA levels.

While many anti-aging enthusiasts are familiar with DHEA, far fewer are likely to be as aware of its metabolite, 7-Keto DHEA, which functions within the body to safely boost immune function and help reduce body fat. The term "7-Keto DHEA" is in fact a brand name for the chemical compound 3-acetyl-7-dehydroepiandrosterone. Human blood levels of both 7-Keto DHEA and DHEA tend to rise and fall in a similar pattern with age: increasing until the twenties, beginning to decline in the thirties, and continuing decline until the levels are reduced by about 50 percent by age fifty. Clinical studies have shown that, as 7-Keto DHEA levels go down in middle age, body weight tends to goes up.

7-Keto DHEA also stimulates weight loss through a process called thermogenesis. This term refers to the creation of heat at a cellular level. The more thermogenesis, the higher the metabolic rate and the more fat that is literally burned up as energy. Studies have also demonstrated that 7-Keto does not accumulate in the body over time and is free of unhealthy side effects.

I have found supplementation with 7-Keto DHEA to be significant. Because 7-Keto DHEA is a natural hormone metabolite, it benefits the body in two ways: (1) it helps restore hormone balance while (2) working internally to melt away those unwanted pounds. I recommend 100 mg of 7-Keto DHEA per day, one capsule every morning.

Go Green

It has already been established that if you live in the United States or other industrialized nations, you are exposed to foreign hormones (xenohormones) every day. These can be absorbed into your system by digestion, inhalation, or direct skin contact. Everyone can take some simple steps to protect themselves and their family. I recommend that you:

- Avoid drinking beverages from plastic bottles. All plastic leaches xenohormones into the environment.
- Avoid microwaving food in plastic containers, and avoid using plastic wrap to cover food for microwaving.
- Wash your food well to rid it of pesticides.

- Throw away all pesticides, herbicides, and fungicides.
- Check product labels for the following chemicals: aliphatic hydrocarbons (n-hexane), halogenated hydrocarbons (carbon tetrachloride, trichloroethylene), alcohols (methanol, ethanol), cyclic hydrocarbons (cyclohexane), esters (ethyl ether), nitrohydrocarbons (ethyl nitrate), ketones (acetone, methylethylketone), glycols (ethylene glycol), aromatic hydrocarbons (benzene), and adehydes (acetaldehyde). Do not buy products if these chemicals are present.
- Check your cosmetics for toxic ingredients and throw them away. Throw away all nail polish and nail polish removers. Note: Most health food stores now stock a variety of organic cosmetics and hair dyes.
- Use organic soaps and toothpastes.
- Don't use fabric softeners, as they put petrochemicals right onto your skin.
- Use only naturally based perfumes. Most perfumes are petrochemical-based.

- Have a good water filter in your home.
- Beware of noxious fumes given off by carpets, copiers, and printers.

Get a Good Night's Sleep

Sleep is one of the most important things you can do every day to support hormone balance. Sleep disturbances are a common symptom of hormone imbalance, but BHRT, most particularly bio-identical progesterone, has been found to promote feelings of relaxation and an ability to sleep through the night. Still, a good night's sleep will only occur if you get into bed, empty your mind, and close your eyes.

Sleep is analogous to the reset button on your computer. When your body "crashes," sleep is the fastest way to reboot. A choice to go to bed later or to do things that interfere with sleep quality or quantity negatively impacts hormone production. To understand how this works, we need to go back to the time of prehistoric humans.

Think of your average prehistoric hunter-gatherer. When the sun went down, he slept; when the sun rose, he woke. His hormones were what allowed his body to know when to sleep and when to wake. In medicine they call this a circadian rhythm; it is the hormonal dance that occurs with the dark-light cycle. Ever since the invention of the lightbulb, our days have been lengthened and our nights have been shortened. Add to this artificial heat and abundant food, and our hormones tell us we are in a perpetual summer. Summertime to a caveman meant eat energy-rich food and get fat for the coming winter. The only problem is, if winter never comes, hormone balance is never restored.

Turning off the lights and sleeping seven to eight hours a night stimulates overall hormone balance. From the caveman's perspective, the body responds as if it has moved into winter. Fat-storing hormones—cortisol and insulin—are lowered, and the equilibrium between the hormones controlling appetite, leptin and ghrelin, is reestablished.

Before I Go

With the help of BHRT and hormone-healthy lifestyle choices, you can restore hormone balance and enjoy the health and vitality that go along with it. I hope you, like thousands of others, will internalize my potentially life-saving advice and move forward to take charge of your hormone health.

C. W. Randolph Jr., M.D.
www.hormonewell.com
www.agelessandwellness.com

Appendix: Resource Listing

The contact information listed in this section is current as of the publication of this book.

The Natural Hormone Institute of America

When Genie James and I cofounded the Natural Hormone Institute of America in 2003, we had two goals in mind. The first was to create a vehicle to educate the medical community and the healthcare consumer about the safety and efficacy of bio-identical hormone therapies. Our second goal was to formalize a business entity to make my over-the-counter bio-identical progesterone cream and other signature products more widely available and to commit a percentage of website profits to support medical research in the field of bio-identical hormone replacement.

To date, I have been overwhelmed by the positive response of many of my physician peers, as well as from interested and educated healthcare consumers. I am grateful that our founding of the Natural Hormone Institute of America appears to be meeting a very real need at the right time.

For more information regarding bio-identical hormone replacement, to discuss scheduling a personal consultation or to purchase the products recommended in this book, go to my interactive website, www.hormone well.com, or contact our office by telephone at 904-694-0039.

Note: we also offer a free biweekly eNewsletter. Just go to www.hormonewell.com to subscribe.

Women In Balance

Women in Balance (WIB) is a national, nonprofit association of women, doctors, health care professionals and organizations dedicated to helping women achieve hormone balance. This organization was founded to educate women and the health care community about hormone imbalance, and its impact on a woman's health and well-being as she ages. It is a non-profit association that is focused on addressing these issues for women, without bias or affiliation.

The WIB website is an outstanding resource. Of particular note is its comprehensive repository of research on BHRT. In addition, for anyone seeking to find a BHRT expert in their area, this website includes a health provider locator tool.

Website: www.womeninbalance.org

Virginia Hopkins

Virginia Hopkins worked closely with Dr. John Lee as the co-author of his groundbreaking books on BHRT. Today, Virginia continues their mission of education regarding the safety and efficacy of natural hormone replacement through her eNewsletter, The Virginia Hopkins Health Watch.

Website: http://www.virginiahopkinstestkits.com

Over-the-Counter Progesterone Creams

You can purchase bio-identical progesterone creams in most health food stores. The good news is that it is available. The bad news is that some products are better than others. The reason for this discrepancy: no regulatory body oversees the production or standardization of product manufacturing for so-called natural products. What this means to the average consumer is that there is great variation among the many OTC progesterone creams on the market today.

While I cannot reveal my exact formula for my Natural Balance Cream, I can outline some of the critical variables that define its excellence and efficacy.

Dr. Randolph's Natural Balance Cream is a bio-identical formulation of progesterone, which means that the molecules of progesterone suspended in the cream have exactly the same molecular structure as those produced by the human body. The body recognizes, receives, and utilizes these molecules. The parent molecule for progesterone comes from a substance known as diosgenin, which is found in soy or Mexican wild yam. Many products on the market today containing soy or Mexican wild yam claim to be a "natural progesterone"; however, until the diosgenin is converted from its original molecular structure, the body will not recognize it. Consequently, soy or Mexican wild yam in its raw state will not generate the same clinical response.

Dr. Randolph's Natural Balance Cream contains the maximum concentration of human-identical progesterone that can be mixed in an over-the-counter product. Some over-the-counter creams have a "little" progesterone in their mix, but not enough to generate a consistent and positive patient response.

The progesterone I use in my formula meets the United States Pharmacopoeia gold standards for quality and purity. In addition, I require that the lab I use to produce Dr. Randolph's Natural Balance Cream compounds my product under strict guidelines approved by the National Association of Compounding Pharmacists. This is not required by law, so not all product manufacturers go to the trouble or expense.

The progesterone molecule in my cream is encased within a liposomal delivery system, which is critical because, as the many layers of the oily globule of liposome melt away like a snowball, the hormones are dispersed continuously through the skin for up to 12 hours. The underlying issue of hormonal imbalance is eliminated, hormonal balance is restored, and my patients have continuous relief of their symptoms throughout the day. In contrast, other over-the-counter progesterone creams are not formulated for sustained release. All the progesterone in these other over-the-counter creams is immediately absorbed through the skin, resulting in a quick spike in progesterone levels and only a temporary relief of symptoms.

I have reviewed several other over-the-counter creams for quality and truth in advertising. These include:

Arbonne International
PhytoProlief and Prolief Natural Balancing Creams
P.O. Box 2488
Laguna Hills, California
Phone: 800-ARBONNE
Website: www.arbonne.com

Emerita
Pro-Gest progesterone cream
621 SW Alder, Suite 900

Portland, Oregon 97205-3627

Phone: 800-648-8211

Website: www.progest.com

The Health and Science Research Institute

Serenity for Women progesterone cream

661 Beville Road, Suite 101

Daytona Beach, Florida 32119

Phone: 888-222-1415

Website: www.health-science.com

HM Enterprises

Happy PMS

2622 Bailey Drive

Norcross, Georgia 30071

Phone: 800-742-4773

Website: www.hmenterprises.com

Life-flo Health Care Products

Progestacare Cream

8146 N. 23rd Avenue, Suite E

Phoenix, Arizona 85021

Phone: 888-999-7440

Website: www.sheld.com/lifeflo

Products of Nature

Natural Woman progesterone cream
54 Danbury Road
Ridgefield, Connecticut 06877
Phone: 800-665-5952
Website: www.pronature.com

Restored Balance Inc.

Restored Balance PMS/Menopausal progesterone cream
42 Meadowbridge Drive SW
Cartersville, Georgia 30120
Phone: 800-865-7499
Website: www.restoredbalanceusa.com

There are many other progesterone creams on the market today that may also contain bio-identical progesterone which I have not reviewed. If you have any doubt or concerns regarding any bio-identical progesterone product, call the company and ask how many milligrams of progesterone per ounce the cream contains.

For the 20 percent of premenopausal women for whom an over-the-counter bio-identical progesterone cream does not completely eliminate their unpleasant symptoms, this can be regarded as a signal that a woman's estrogen or testosterone levels have also begun to decline. At this time, a blood work or saliva test may be an appropriate next step to evaluate the current ratio of all three sex hormones.

On my website I offer a viable option for those women or men who believe or have evidence that the balance of their other hormones has shifted and requires treatment. Go to http://www.hormonewell.com/hormoneconsultation.html to learn more about how you can obtain a comprehensive hormone level profile via a saliva test, and then schedule a one-on-one telephone consultation with me or one of my personally trained nurse practitioners.

Personal Hormone-Level Profile

Blood Testing

MyMedLab is a leading provider of state-of-the-art laboratory testing. MyMedLab works directly with nationally renowned physicians, like myself, to develop specific groups of laboratory tests called Profiles. Blood analysis of hormone levels are available direct to consumers without a doctor's visit or appointment at more than two thousand collection sites across the United States.

To learn more about MyMedLab and the C. W. Randolph, M.D., Hormone Hell-Well Profiles, contact:

MyMedLab Inc.
2401 South Jackson
Joplin, Missouri 64804
Phone: 888-696-3352
Website: www.mymedlab.com

Salivary and Blood Spot Testing

ZRT Laboratory's state-of-the-art saliva and capillary blood spot testing technology allows for accurate measurement of a broad array of hormones and detection of existing hormone imbalance. Dr. David Zava, the founder of ZRT Laboratory, is also the coauthor with John R. Lee, M.D., of *What Your Doctor May Not Tell You About Breast Cancer.*

Saliva Testing

Convenient, accurate, and inexpensive home collection, Saliva Testing provides a true picture of the bioavailable levels of steroid hormones.

Capillary Blood Spot Testing

Capillary Blood Spot Testing offers an easy, finger-stick alternative to blood draws in the doctor's office.

Combination Saliva and Capillary Blood Spot Testing

Combines both saliva and capillary blood spot test materials in an all-in-one test kit for easy home collection of the major hormone groups—reproductive, adrenal, and thyroid—on the same day at the optimal time.

To initiate a relationship with ZRT or to find out more, contact:

ZRT Laboratories
1815 NW 169th Place, Suite 5050
Beaverton, Oregon 97006
Phone: 503-466-2445
Fax: 503-466-1636
Website: http://www.salivatest.com

Locating a Physician

Again, Women In Balance (WIB) now includes a health provider locator tool on their website, www.womeninbalance.org.

In addition, a local compounding pharmacist can be an excellent resource for locating a physician in your area who is knowledgeable about BHRT. If you need help finding a compounding pharmacy in your area, contact one of the two organizations listed below.

The International Academy of Compounding Pharmacists (IACP)
P.O. Box 1365
Sugar Land, Texas 7787
Phone: 281-933-8400
Fax: 281-495-0602
Website: http://www.iacprx.org

IACP was established in 1991 as Professionals and Patients for Customized Care (P2C2). In 1996, P2C2 changed its name to IACP in an effort to broaden its scope and recognize changes in the profession. Today, the IACP has more than eighteen hundred members internationally, serving pharmacists, physicians, students, and patients.

Professional Compounding Centers of America (PCCA)
9901 S. Wilcrest Drive
Houston, Texas 77099
Phone: 877-798-3224
Fax: 877-765-1422
Website: http://www.pccarx.com

PCCA provides independent pharmacists with a complete support system from compounding unique dosage forms. Founded in 1981, PCCA has more than three thousand pharmacist members located throughout the United States, Canada, Australia, Europe, and New Zealand. On an average, PCCA's consulting department answers more than five hundred calls per day, providing members with comprehensive technical support.

COMPOUNDING PHARMACIES

Throughout this book, I'm sure you have noticed a recurring theme that one size does not fit all when it comes to hormone replacement. As you learned in chapter 5, compounding pharmacies can be a resource for physicians who are interested in moving away from the use of synthetic HRT, but do not have the experience or training in new areas such as the use of saliva testing and the subsequent prescription of bio-identical hormones. Today's compounding pharmacies can produce literally whatever the doctor orders. A physician can work with a compounding pharmacy to develop personalized prescriptions of bio-identical hormones to meet the unique needs of each individual patient.

If you have never before heard of or used a compounding pharmacy, here are some key facts that you may want to consider:

- Every compounding pharmacy is licensed and inspected by the State Pharmacy Board.
- Compounding pharmacists are educated and trained to provide information regarding the formulation of bio-identical hormones; they can reassure, educate, and provide physicians with safe dosage guidelines for bio-identical hormone supplementation.

- All materials used in compounding formulations are subject to FDA inspection and the agency's Good Manufacturing Procedures code.

All pharmacies associated with the previously described compounding pharmacy organizations, PCCA and IACP, meet this criteria. In addition, there are two other national compounding pharmacies that I often recommend to physicians:

College Pharmacy
3505 Austin Bluffs Parkway, Suite 101
Colorado Springs, Colorado 80918
Phone: 800-888-9358
Website: http://www.collegepharmacy.com

Women's International Pharmacy
2 Marsh Court
Madison, Wisconsin 53718
Phone: 800-279-5708
Website: http://www.womensinternational.com

Biopharmaceutical Companies

I am grateful to report that there are now several specialty biopharmaceutical companies dedicating resources and dollars to developing proprietary bio-identical/bio-identical hormone products. The following is a list of some of the products with which I am currently familiar and prescribe in my own practice. Each of these has been approved by the FDA.

Bio-Identical Estradiol

Divigel
EstroGel
Estrace
Estrasorb
Evamist

Bio-Identical Progesterone

Prochieve
Prometrium

Bio-Identical Testosterone

Androgel
Testoderm

Grocery Stores

Because of growing consumer demand, I am excited to report that almost every grocery store in the nation stocks some organic foods. Still, my hat goes off to Whole Foods Market. Founded in 1980 as one small store in Austin, Texas, Whole Foods Market is now the world's leading retailer of natural and organic foods, with 270 stores in North America and the United Kingdom. To find a Whole Foods Market near you, go to www.wholefoodsmarket.com.

Organic Food Websites

Many people initially complain that buying organic is too expensive. Organic foods can be pricey if you just shop in your supermarket, but you probably have a lot more choices for organic food in your community than you realize. To find a source of organic foods near you or to order online, check out the following websites: www.organicfoods.com, www.organicconsumer.org, www.eatwell.com, and www.diamondorganics.com. Also, local farmers markets can be a great source for organic foods, often at lower prices than you will pay in the supermarket or health food store.

Favorite Brands

Vitamins and Supplements

When I opened my first Natural Medicine Store, I stocked the shelves with natural products from a variety of manufacturers. It was not long before the difference in my patients' and customers' responses signaled to me that not all product manufacturers could be trusted. According to a recent survey conducted by ConsumerLab.com, a product-certification company, one out of four of nearly 1,000 supplements tested has quality problems. These include contamination or a failure to include an ingredient listed on the label.

As I became aware of the discrepancy between manufacturers, I drew on my professional training and experience as a compounding pharmacist to establish criteria which would ensure that any products in my shop and on my website were safe and effective.

My criterion for my own private-label products was and is simple yet unnegotiable: *quality and truth in labeling*, which for my own private-labeled line—as well as other natural health product lines that I carry—means that I require stringent guidelines for their manufacturing process. These guidelines include:

- Raw materials testing
- Potency testing
- Product traceability
- Purity testing
- Product freshness
- Microbiology testing

The bottom line is truth in packaging. People have the right to know what they are putting into their body, and they deserve to get the amount of active ingredient for which they are paying.

To order Dr. Randolph's products online, go to www.hormonewell.com/shop_online.htm.

Life Extension is a source for vitamins and supplements in which I have the highest level of confidence. This company's manufacturing standards ensure exceptional purity and quality. The company provides access for its members to a toll-free phone line where they can speak with holistic health advisors and medical doctors about their individual health concerns. In addition to its natural product offerings, Life Extension publishes a fantastic monthly magazine. For more information on Life Extension, go to www.lef.org or call 1-800-226-2370.

Recommended Reading

As I have mentioned throughout the book, many other physician pioneers have helped lay a foundation of learning and knowledge in the study of bio-identical hormone therapy. I have the following books in my personal library. Each author offers the reader the benefit of additional information and another perspective. Please note that these resources are not prioritized by perceived merit, but are listed in alphabetical order according to author:

Lee, John R. *Natural Progesterone: The Multiple Role of a Remarkable Hormone.* Sebastopol, CA: BLL Publishing, 1993.

———, with Jesse Hanley and Virginia Hopkins. *What Your Doctor May Not Tell You About Perimenopause.* New York: Warner Books, 1999.

Lee, John R., with Virginia Hopkins. *What Your Doctor May Not Tell You About Menopause.* New York: Warner Books, 1996.

Lee, John R., with David Zava and Virginia Hopkins. *What Your Doctor May Not Tell You About Breast Cancer: How Hormone Balance Can Help Save Your Life.* New York: Warner Books, 2002.

Leonetti, Helene B. *Menopause: A Spiritual Renaissance—What You Can Do to Empower Your Life from Someone Who's Been There and Done It.* Carson City, NJ: Bridger House, 2002.

Northrup, Christiane. *The Wisdom of Menopause: Creating Physical and Emotional Health and Healing During the Change.* New York: Bantam Books, 2001.

———. *Women's Bodies, Women's Wisdom: Creating Physical and Emotional Health and Healing.* New York: Bantam Books, 1994.

Schwartz, Erika. *The Hormone Solution.* New York: Warner Books, 2002.

Seaman, Barbara. *The Doctors' Case Against the Pill.* Alameda, CA: Hunter House, 1969.

Shulman, Neil, and Kim S. Edmunds. *Healthy Transitions: A Woman's Guide to Perimenopause, Menopause & Beyond.* New York: Prometheus Books, 2004.

Somers, Suzanne. *Breakthrough: Eight Steps to Wellness.* New York: Crown Publishers, 2008.

———. *The Sexy Years: Discover the Hormone Connection—The Secret to Fabulous Sex, Great Health, and Vitality for Women and Men.* New York: Crown Publishers, 2004.

Stephenson, Kenna. *Awakening Athena: Resilience, Restoration, and Rejuvenation for Women.* Tyler, TX: Heart Health and Mind Institute, 2004

Taylor, Eldred, and Ava Bell-Taylor. *Are Your Hormones Making You Sick?* Physicians Natural Medicine, 2000.

Whitaker, Julian. *Dr. Whitaker's Guide to Natural Hormone Replacement.* Potomac, MD: Phillips Publishing, 1999.

Wilson, James L. *Adrenal Fatigue.* Petaluma, CA: Smart Publications, 2003.

Wright, Jonathan V., and John Morgenthaler. *Natural Hormone Replacement for Women over 45.* Petaluma, CA: Smart Publications, 1997.

The Best Resource: Yourself

As I end this book, I want to take a moment to remind each reader that no one can tell you what is right for you or for your health. I encourage you to listen, read, ask questions, and seek out others who feel that they are in hormone hell to share information and experiences. I applaud you for seeking additional medical counsel to better understand your options and choices for hormone replacement. Once you have the data in hand, I believe that the most important thing you can do is to get quiet and listen to your heart. Within each of us is the wisdom we need to make the right decisions.

Notes

Chapter 1: Decades of Desperate Women Dangerously Duped

1. Susan Benedict and Jane M. Georges, "Nurses and the sterilization experiments of Auschwitz: a postmodernist perspective," *Nursing Inquiry* 13, no. 4 (2006): 277–88.
2. Robert Koenig, "Reopening the Darkest Chapter in German Science," *Science*, June 3, 2000.
3. Barbara Seaman, *The Greatest Experiment Ever Performed on Women* (New York: Hyperion, 2003), 28.
4. Ibid., 212.
5. Tobias Milrood, "The Rise and Fall of Hormone Therapy," citing Writing Group for the Women's Health Initiative Investigators, "Risks and Benefits of Estrogen Plus Progestin in Healthy Postmenopausal Women," *Journal of the American Medical Association* 288 (2002): 321.
6. Sally A. Shumaker, Claudine Legault, Stephen R. Rapp, et al., for the WHIMS Investigators, "Estrogen Plus Progestin and the Incidence of Dementia and mild Cognitive Impairment in Postmenopausal Women," *Journal of the American Medical Association* 289, no. 20 (2003).

7. Rowan T. Chlebowski, Susan L. Hendrix, Robert D. Langer, et al., for the WHI Investigators, "Influence of Estrogen Plus Progestin on Breast Cancer and Mammography in Healthy Postmenopausal Women," *Journal of the American Medical Association* 289, no. 24 (2003); C. L. Dillis and J. S. Schreiman, "Change in Mammographic Breast Density Associated with the Use of Depo-Provera," *Breast Journal* 9, no. 4 (2003): 312–15.

8. Tomas Riman, Paul W. Dickman, Stafan Nilsson, et al., "Hormone Replacement Therapy and the Risk of Invasive Epithelial Ovarian Cancer in Swedish Women," National Cancer Institute, April 2002.

9. M. Ravdin, K. A. Cronin, N. Howlander, et al., "The Decrease in Breast Cancer Incidence in 2003 in the United States," *New England Journal of Medicine* 356, no. 16 (2007).

Chapter 2—Bio-Identical Hormone Replacement Therapy (BHRT): A Safe and Effective Alternative

1. North American Menopause Society, "Menopause Is the Beginning of a New, Fulfilling Stage of Life, the NAMS 1997 Menopause Survey Shows," *Journal of the North American Menopause Society* 5, no. 4 (1997).

2. Christiane Northrup, *The Wisdom of Menopause* (New York: Bantam Books, 2001), 141.

3. Loyd V. Allen Jr., "Estriol: Women's Choice vs. A Manufacturer's Greed," *International Journal of Medicine* 12, no. 4 (2008): 289.

4. Deborah Grady, Bruce Ettinger, Anna N. A. Tosteson, Alice Pressman, Judith L. Macer, "Predators of Difficulty When Discontinuing Postmenopausal Hormone Therapy," *Obstetrics and Gynecology* 102, no. 6 (2003): 1233–39.

Chapter 5—It's Not Just Your Age . . . It's Your Life

1. John R. Lee and Virginia Hopkins, "Part II: Xenohormones in Your Environment: Rounding Up the Usual Suspects—When It Comes to Chemicals, Assume the Worst and When in Doubt, Don't," *John R. Lee Medical Letter,* http://www.virginiahopkinstestkits.com/xeno hormoneII.html (accessed October 27, 2008).
2. Katherine M. Shea, "Pediatric Exposure and Potential Toxicity of Phthalate Plasticizers," *Pediatrics* 111 (2003): 1467–74.
3. http://www.womentowomen.com/menopause/estrogendominance.aspx.
4. Warren Cornwall and Keith Ervin, "Hormonal Chemicals May Be Imperiling Fish," *Seattle Times,* April 1, 2007.

Chapter 6—More Than Uncomfortable: How Hormone Imbalance Impacts Health and Mortality

1. Cheryl L. Rock, Shirley W. Flatt, Gail A. Laughlin, et al., "Reproductive Steroid Hormones and Recurrence-Free Survival in Women with a History of Breast Cancer," *Cancer Epidemiology Biomarkers and Prevention* 17 (2008): 614–20.
2. John R. Lee, "Hormone Balance for Men: What Your Doctor May Not Tell You about Prostate Health and Natural Hormone Supplementation," 2003.
3. R. A. Whitmer, D. R. Gustafson, E. Barrett-Connor, M. N. Haan, E. P. Gunderson, and K. Yaffe, "Central Obesity and Increased Risk of Dementia More Than Three Decades Later," *Neurology* 71 (2008): 1057–64.
4. Cuilin Zhang, Kathryn M. Rexrode, Rob M. van Dam, Tricia Y. Li, and Frank B. Hu, "Abdominal Obesity and the Risk of All-Cause Cardiovascular, and Cancer Mortality: Sixteen Years of Follow-up in U.S. Women," *American Heart Association* 117 (2008): 1658–67.

5. Beverley Balkau, John E. Deanfield, Jean-Pierre Despres, et al., "International Day for the Evaluation of Abdominal Obesity (IDEA): A Study of Waist Circumference, Cardiovascular Disease, and Diabetes Mellitus in 168,000 Primary Care Patients in 63 Countries," *American Heart Association* 116 (2007): 1942–51.

6. Kay-Tee Khaw, Mitch Dowsett, Elizabeth Folkerd, et al., "Endogenous Testosterone and Mortality Due to All Causes, Cardiovascular Disease, and Cancer in Men: European Prospective Investigation into Cancer in Norfolk (EPIC-Norfolk) Prospective Population Study," *American Heart Association* 116 (2007): 2694–2707.

7. Eewa A. Jankowska, Bartosz Biel, Jocek Majda, et al., "Anabolic Deficiency in Men with Chronic Heart Failure: Prevalence and Detrimental Impact on Survival," *American Heart Association* 114 (2006): 1829–37.

Chapter 7—Step 1: Start with Bio-Identical Progesterone

1. K. Stephenson, P. F. Neuenschwander, A. K. Kurdowska, B. Pinson, and C. Price, "Progesterone Effects on Menopausal Symptoms and on Thrombotic, Anticoagulant, and Inflammatory Factors in Postmenopausal Women," *International Journal of Pharmaceutical Compounding* 12, no.4 (2008): 295–304.

2. A. Fournier, F. Berrino, E. Riboli, V. Avenel, and F. Clavel-Chapelon, "Breast Cancer Risk in Relation to Different Types of Hormone Replacement Therapy in the E3N-EPIC Cohort," *International Journal of Cancer* 114 (2005): 448–54.

3. N. C. Jones, D. Constantine, M. J. W. Prior, P. G. Morris, C. A. Marsden, and S. Murphy, "The neuroprotective effect of progesterone after traumatic brain injury in male mice is independent of both the inflammatory response and growth factor expression," *European Journal of Neuroscience* 21 (2005): 1547–1554; D. G. Stein,"Brain damage, sex hormones and recovery: a new role for pro-

gesterone and estrogen?" *Trends in Neurosciences* 24, no.7 (2001): 386–391; D. W. Wright, A. L. Kellerman, V. S. Hertzberg, et al., "ProTECT: a randomized clinical trial of progesterone for acute traumatic brain injury," Annals of Emergency Medicine 51 (2008): 164–172.

4. R. Kaaks, F. Berrino, T. Key, et al., "Serum Sex Steroids in Premenopausal Women and Breast Cancer Risk within the European Prospective Investigation into Cancer and Nutrition (EPIC)," *Journal of the National Cancer Institute* 97 (2005): 755–65; Fournier, Berrino, Riboli, Avenel, and Clavel-Chapelon, "Breast Cancer Risk"; K. J. Chang et al., "Influences of Percutaneous Administration of Estradiol and Progesterone on Human Breast Epithelial Cycle in Vivo," *Fertility and Sterility* 63 (1995): 785–91; L. D. Cowan et al., "Breast Cancer Incidence in Women with a History of Progesterone Deficiency," *American Journal of Epidemiology* 114 (1981): 209–17.

5. I. J. Laidlaw and R. B. Clarke, "The Proliferation of Normal Cell Tissue Implanted into Athymic Nude Mice Is Stimulated by Estrogen, but Not by Progesterone," *Endocrinology* 136 (1995): 164–71; Giuseppe M. C. Rosano, Carolyn M. Webb, Sergio Chierchia, et al., "Natural Progesterone, but Not Medroxyprogesterone Acetate, Enhances the Beneficial Effect of Estrogen on Exercise-Induced Myocardial Ischemia in Postmenopausal Women," *Journal of the American College of Cardiology* 36 (2000): 2154; C. Molinari, A. Battaglia, E. Grossini, et al., "Effect of Progesterone on Peripheral Blood Flow in Prepubertal Female Anesthetized Pigs," *Journal of Vascular Research* 38 (2001): 569–77; J. K. Williams, E. K. Honore, S. A. Washburn, et al., "Effects of Hormone Replacement Therapy on Reactivity of Artherosclerotic Coronary Arteries in Cynomolgus Monkeys," *Journal of American College of Cardiology* 224 (1994): 1757–61.

6. Morris Noteloviz, *Stand Tall: Every Woman's Guide to Preventing and Treating Osteoporosis* (Gainesville, FL: Triad Publishing Company, 1998).

7. W. S. Maxson, "The Use of Progesterone in the Treatment of PMS," *Clinical Obstetrics and Gynecology* 30 (1987): 465–77.

8. Lorraine A. Fitzpatrick, Cindy Pace, and Brinda Wiita, "Comparison of Regimens Containing Oral Micronized Progesterone or Medroxyprogesterone Acetate on Quality of Life in Postmenopausal Women: A Cross-Sectional Survey," *Journal of Women's Health and Gender-Based Medicine* 9, no. 4 (2000): 381–87.

References

Chapter 1

American College of Obstetricians and Gynecologists. Risk of breast cancer with estrogen-progestin replacement therapy. *Int J Gynaecol Obstet.* 2002; 76: 333—335.

Susan Benedict and Jane M. Georges Nurses and the sterilization experiments of Auschwitz: a postmodernist perspective. *Nursing Inquiry*— 2006; 13(4):277—288

Beral V, Colwell—Randomized trial of high doses of stilbestrol and ethisterone in pregnancy: long-term follow-up of mothers. *Brit Med J* 1980; 281:1098—1011

Bibbo M, Haenszel WM, Wied GL, Hubby M, Herbst AL.—A twenty-five year follow-up study of women exposed to diethylstilbestrol during pregnancy. *New England Journal of Medicine* 1978; 298(14): 763–7

Brian DD, Tilley BC, Labarthe DR, O'Fallon WM, Noller KL, Kurland LT.—Breast cancer in DES-exposed mothers—absence of association. *Mayo Clin* Pro 1980; 55:89–93

Braun MM, Ahlbom A, Floderus B, Brinton LA, Hoover RN.—Effect of twinship in incidence of cancer of the testis, breasts, and other sites [*Sweden*]. Cancer Causes Control 1995; 6:519–24.

B.M. Caldwell & R.I. Watson, An Evaluation of Psychologic Effects of Sex Hormone Administration in Aged Women: Results of Therapy after Six Months, 7 J. *GERONTOLOGY* 228 (1952)

Rowan T. Chlebowski, MD, PhD; Susan L Hendrix, DO; Robert D Langer, MD, MPH; Marcia L Stefanick, PhD; Margery Gass, MD; Dorothy Lane, MD, MPH; Rebecca J. Rodabough, MS; Mary Ann Gilligan, MD, MPH; Michele G. Cyr, MD; Cynthia A Thomson, PhD, RD; Janardan Khandekar, MD; Helen Petrovitch, MD; Anne McTiernan, MDk, PhD: for the WHI Investigators—Influence of Estrogen Plus Progestin on Breast Cancer and mammography in Healthy Postmenopausal Women." *The Journal of the American Medical Association* Vol. 289 No. 24, June 25, 2003

Collaborative Group on Hormonal Factors in Breast Cancer. Breast cancer and hormone replacement therapy: collaborative reanalysis of data from 51 epidemiological studies of 52, 705 women with breast cancer and 108, 411 women without breast cancer. *Lancet* 1997; 350:1047–1059.

Dillis C.L.; Schreiman J.s.—Change in Mammographic Breast Density Associated with the Use of Depo-Provera."—*The Breast Journal,* 2003; 9(4):312–315

Peter H. Gann and Monica Morrow. Combined hormone therapy and breast cancer: A single-edged Sword. *JAMA* 2003; 289(24):3304–3306

Gavin, N., Thorp, J., and Oshfeldt, R.—Determinants of hormone replacement therapy duration among postmenopausal women with intact uteri. *Menopause,* 2001; 8:377–383.

Gillson, G. R., and Zava, D. T.—Perspective on Hormone Replacement for Women: Picking up the pieces after the Women's Health Initiative Trial. *International Journal of Pharmaceutical Compounding,* 2003; 7(4):250.

Greendale GA, Reboussin BA, sie A, et al. Effects of estrogen and estrogen-progestin on mammographic parenchymal density. *Ann Intern Med.* 1999;130:262–269Hadjimichael OC, Meigs JW, Falcier FW, Thompson WD, Flannery JT. Cancer risk among women exposed to exogenous estroens during pregnancy. *J Natl Cancer Inst* 1984; 73(4)831–4

Hadjimichael OC, Meigs JW, Falcier FW, Thompson WD, Flannery JT—Cancer risk among women exposed to exogenous estrogens during pregnancy. *J Natl Cancer Inst* 1984; 4(4):831–4

Jennifer Hays et al., Effects of Estrogen Plus Progestin on Health—Related Quality of Life, 348 *New Eng J Med* 1893 2003

Herbst AL, Poskanzer DC, Robboy SJ, Friedlander I, Scully RE.—A prospective comparison of exposed female offspring with unexposed controls. *N Engl J Med* 1975; 292(7):334–9

Lars Holmberg, Ole-Erik Iversen, Carl Mgnus Rudenstam, Mats Hammar, Eero Kumpulainen, Janusz Jaskiewicz, Jacek Jassem, Daria Dobaczewska, Hans E. Fjosne, Octavio Peralta, Rodrigo Arriagda, Marit Holmqvist, and Johanna Maenpa On behalf of the HABITS Study Group.—Increased risk of recurrence after hormone replacement therapy in breast cancer survivors. *J Natl Cancer Inst*, 2008; 100:475–482

Christopher I. Li, Kathleen E. Malone, Peggy L. Porter, Noel S. Weiss, Mei-Tzu C. Tang, Kara L. Cushing-Haugen and Janet R. Daling—Relationship between long duration and different regimens of hormone therapy and risk of breast cancer. *JAMA*. 2003; 289(24): 3254–3263

Khan SA, MA Rogers, KK Khurana, MM MEguid and PJ Numann Estrogen receptor expression in benign breast epithelium and breast cancer risk *J Natl Cancer Inst* 1992;84:1575–1582

Robert Koenig Reopening the Darkest Chapter in German Science.—*Science Magazine*, 3 June 2000

James V. Lacey Jr. et al.,—Menopausal Hormone Replacement Therapy and Risk of Ovarian Cancer, 288 *JAMA* 334 2002

Manjer J, Malina J, Berglund G, et al. Increased incidence of small and well-differentiated breast tumours in post-menopausal women following hormone replacement therapy. *Int J Cancer*. 2001;92:919–922

McCarthy Eliza Estrogen Uncovered Have women been the unwitting victims of the medical establishment's experiment with hormones?—*Slate* 2003

Meara J, Vessey M, Fairweather DV. A randomized double-blind controlled trial of the value of diethylstilbestrol therapy in pregnancy: 35 years follow-up of mothers and their offspring. *Brit J Obstet Gynecol* 1989;96(5):620–2

Tobias Millrod Writing Group for the Women's Health Initiative Investigators, Risks and Benefits of Estrogen Plus Progestin in Healthy Postmenopausal Women, 288 *The Journal of the American Medical Association* 321 (2002

Mosby.—*Human Pharmacology*, Third Edition. Mosby-Year Book, Inc., St. Louis, Missouri, 1998

Muller-Hill Benno Genetics of susceptibility to tuberculosis: Mengele's experiments in Auschwitz *Nature Reviews Genetics* 2001 2:631–634

National Institutes of Health News Release. (July 9, 2002). NLHBI Stops Trial of Estrogen Plus Progestin Due to Increased Breast Cancer Risk, Lack of Overall Benefit.

Prentice et al.—Conjugated equine estrogens and breast cancer risk in the Women's Health Initiative clinical trial and observational study. *Am J Epidemion* 2008;167:1407–1415

Prentice et al.—Estrogen plus progestin therapy and breast cancer in recently postmenopausal women. *Am JEpidemion* 2008;167:1207–1216

Ravdin M, Cronin KA, Howlander N, Berg CD, Chlebowski RT, Feuer EJ, Edwards BK, Berry DA.—The Decrease in Breast Cancer Incidence in 2003 in the United States." *New England Journal of Medicine* Vol. 356, No. 16, April 19, 2007

Tomas Riman, Paul W. Dickman, Stafan Nilsson, Nestor Correia, Hans Nordlinger, Cecilia M. Magnusson, Elisabete Weiderpass, and Ingermar R. Persson—Hormone Replacement therapy and the Risk of Invasive Epithelial Ovarian Cancer in Swedish Women *–National Cancer Institute,* April 2002

Ross RK, Paganini-Hill A, Wan PC, Pike MC. Effect of hormone replacement therapy on breast cancer risk. *J. Natl Cancer Inst.* 2000;92:328–332

Rossouw JE, Anderson GL, Prentice RL, et al, for Writing Group for the Women's Health Initiative. Risks and benefits of estrogen plus progestin in healthy postmenopausal women: principal results from the Women Health Initiative. *JAMA* 2002;288: 321–333.

Schechter D. (1999). Estrogen, progesterone, and mood. *Journal of Gender-Specific Medicine* 1999; 2:29–36.

Barbara Seaman, *The Greatest Experiment Ever Performed on Woman,* Hyperion 2003 p. 28, p. 212

Sally A. Shumaker, Ph; Claudine Legault, PhD; Stephen R. Rapp, PhD.; Leon Thal, MD; Robert B. Wallace, MD; Judithe K. Ockene, PhD,k MEd; Susan L Hendrix, DO; Beverly N. Jones III, MD; Annlouise R. Assaf, PhD; Rebecca D. Jackson, MD; Jane Morley Kotchen MD, MPH; Sylvia W Sassertheil-Smoller, PhD; Jean Wactawski-Wende, PhD; for the WHIMS Investigators—Estrogen Plus Progestin and the Incidence of Dementia and mild Cognitive Impairment in Postmenopausal Women." *The Journal of the American Medical Association* Vol. 289 No. 20, may 28, 2003

Schairer C, Lubin J, Troisi R, et al. Menopausal estrogen and estrogen-progestin replacement therapy and breast cancer risk. *JAMA* 2000;283:485–494

Sally A Shumaker et al., Estrogen Plus Progestin and the Incidence of Dementia and Mild Cognitive Impairment in Postmenopausal Women, 289 *JAMA* 2651 (2003)

Darcy V. Spicer, Giske Ursin, Yuri R. Parisky, John G. Pearce, Donna Shoupe, Anne Pike, and Malcolm C. Pike. Changes in Mammographic densities induced by a hormonal contraceptive designed to reduce breast cancer risk. J Natl Cancer Inst, 1994;86:431–436

The Women's Health Initiative Study Group. Design of the Women's Health Initiative clinical trial and observational study. *Control Clin Trials.* 1998;19:61–109

The Writing Group for the Women's Health Initiative. (2002). Risks and benefits of estrogen plus progestin in healthy post-menopausal women. *The Journal of the American Medical Association,* 288:321–333.

Titus-Ernstoff L, Hatch EE, Hoover RN, Palmer J, Greenber Er, Ricker W, et. Al. Long-term cancer risk in women given diethylstilbestrol (DES) during pregnancy. *BR J Cancer* 2001;84:126–33

Vessey MP, Fairweather DVI, Norman-Smith B, Buckley J. A randomized double blind controlled trial of the value of diethystillbestrol therapy in pregnancy: Long term follow-up of mothers and offspring *Brit J Obstet Gynecol* 1983;90:1007–17

Whiteman MK, Cui Y, Flaws JA, et al. Media coverage of women's health issues: is there a bias in the reporting of an association between hormone replacement therapy and breast cancer? J *Womens Health Gend Based Med.* 2001;10:571–577.

Robert A. Wilson, The Roles of Estrogen and Progesterone in Breast and Genital Cancer, 182 *JAMA* 327 1962

Wingard DL, Turiel J. Long-term effects of exposure to diethylstilbestrol. West J Med 1988;149(5):551–4

Jonathan V. Wright, M.D. and John Morgenthaler. (1997). *Natural Hormone Replacement,* Smart Publications, CA 23.

Wright JV—Comparative measurements of serum estriol, estradiol, and E1 in non-pregnant, premenopausal women; A preliminary investigation. *Alternative Medicine Review ;4,* 1999:266270.

Peter J. Zandi et al., Hormone Replacement Therapy and Incidence of Alzheimer's Disease in Older Women: The Cache County Study, 288 *JAMA* 2123 2002

Chapter 2

Marcia Angell, MD—The Truth About the Drug Companies—*How They Deceive us and What To Do About It*—Random House, Inc. 2004

Bagis T, Gokcel A, Zeyneloglu HB, Tarim E, Kilicdag EB, Haydardedeoglu B. The effects of short-term medroxyprogesterone acetate and micronized progesterone on glucose metabolism and lipid profiles in patients with polycystic ovary syndrome: a prospective randomized study. *J Clin Endocrinol Metab* 2002 Oct;87(10):4536–40

Boothby, Lisa A PharmD 1; Doering Paul L. MS 2; Kipersztok, Simon MD 3—Bioidentical hormone therapy: a review. *Menopause* 2004; 11(3):356–367

Boothby LAPD, PL; Doering, S Kipersztok—Bioidentical hormone therapy: a review. Menopause 2004; 11(3):356–367

Campagnoli C, Clavel-Chapelon F, Kaaks R, Peris C, Berrino F. Progestins and progesterone in hormone replacement therapy and the risk of breast cancer. *J Steroid Biochem Mol Biol* 2005; 96(2):95–108

De Lignieres B. Effects of progestrogens on the postmenopausal breast. *Climacteric* 2002; 5(3):229–35

Fournier A, Berrino F, Riboli E, Avenel V, Clavel-Chapelon F. Breast Cancer risk in relation to different types of replacement therapy in the E3N-EPIC cohort. *Int J Cancer* 2005; 114(3)448–54

Deborah Grady, MD, MPH, Bruce Ettinger, MD; Anna Tosteson, ScD; Alice Pressman, MS; Judith L. Macer, BSc; "Preditors of difficulty when discontinuing postmenopausal hormone therapy." *Obstetrics & Gynecology* 2003 102(6):1233–1239

Graham JD, and Clarke CL.—Physiological action of progesterone in target tissues. *Endocrine Reviews 18* 1997; 4:502–519.

Lee, John R. MD. *Natural Progesterone—The Multiple Roles of a Remarkable Hormone* BLL Publishing, 1993

Lee, John R. MD, David Zava PhD & Virginia Hopkins *What your Doctor May NOT Tell You About Breast Cancer*—Warner Books 2002

Lee, John R. MD & Virginia Hopkins *What your Doctor May NOT Tell You About Menopause*—Hachette Book Group USA 1996

Lee, John R. MD & Virginia Hopkins *What your Doctor May NOT Tell You About PreMenopause*—Hachette Book Group USA 1999

Leonetti HB, Landes J, Steinberg D, Anasti JN. Topical progesterone cream as an alternative progestin in hormone therapy. *Altern There Health Med* 2005; 11(6):36–38.

Lobo RA. Progestogen metabolism. *J Reprod Med* 1999 Feb;44(2 Suppl):148–52

Lowe, G.D.O.—Hormone replacement therapy: prothrombotic vs. protective effects *Pathophysiology of Haemostasis and Thrombosis* 2002 32(5–6):329–332

Loyd V. Allen, Jr., PhD, RPh—"Estriol: Women's Choice vs. A Manufacturer's Greed." *International Journal of Medicine* 2008: 12(4) p. 289

"Menopause is the Beginning of a new, fulfilling stage of life, The NAMS 1997 Menopause Survey Shows" *The Journal of the North American Menopause Society*, Volume 5 Issue 4.

Moskowitz D—A comprehensive review of the safety and efficacy of bioidentical hormones for the management of menopause and related health risks. *Altern Med Rev* 2006; 11(3):208–23

Christiane Northrup, MD, *The Wisdom of Menopause,* Bantam Books 2001 p. 141

Schechter D. (1999). Estrogen, progesterone, and mood. *Journal of Gender-Specific Medicine ;2,* 29–36

Stanczyk FZ. All progestins are not created equal. *Steroids* 2003; 68:879–90

Wright JV. (1999). Comparative measurements of serum estriol, estradiol, and E1 in non-pregnant, premenopausal women; A preliminary investigation. *Alternative Medicine Review, (4)* , 266270.

Chapter 3

Barrett-Connor E, Grady D, Stefanik ML. The rise and fall of menopausal hormone therapy. *Ann Rev Public Health* 2005; 26:115–40

Borkin, Michael N.M.D.—The Endocrine System and the Female Cycle. *Alternative Medicine Magazine* 2000 #37

Constanti, A.; Bartke, A; and Khardori, R.—Basic Endocrinology for Students of Pharmacy and Allied Clinical Health Sciences. Amsterdam: *Harwood Academic Publishers,* 1998

Friel PN, Hinchcliffe C, Wright JV.—Hormone replacement with estradiol: conventional oral doses result in excessive exposure to estrone. *Altern Med Rev.* 2005 Mar;10(1):36–41

Granberg S, Eurenius K, Lindgren R, Wilhelmsson L. The effects of oral estriol on the endometrium in postmenopausal women. *Maturitas* 2002 Jun 25;42(2):149–56

Hargrove, Joel T. MD, Wayne S. Maxson, MD, Anne Colston Wentz, MD and Lonnie S.l Burnett, MD—Menopausal Hormone Replacement Therapy with Continuous Daily oral Micronized Estradiol and Progesterone—*Obstetrics & Gynecology* 1989;73:606–612

Hasson, H. (1993). Cervical removal at hysterectomy for benign disease. *Journal of Reproductive Medicine,* 1993; 58(10):781–789

Haspels AA, Luisi M, Kicovic PM. Endocrinological and clinical investigations in post-menopausal women following administration of vaginal cream containing estriol. *Maturitas* 1981 Dec;3(3–4):321–7

Ho JY, Chen MJ, Sheu WH, Yi YC, Tsai AC, Guu HF, Ho ES. Differential effects of oral conjugated equine estrogen and transdermal estrogen on atherosclerotic vascular disease risk markers and endothelial function in healthy postmenopausal women. *Hum Reprod* 2006; 21(10):2715–20

Jarupanich T, Lamlertkittikul S, Chandeying V. Efficacy, safety and acceptability of a seven-day, transdermal estradiol patch for estrogen replacement therapy. *J Med Assoc Thai* . 2003 Sep;86(9):836–45

Lee, John R. M.D.—*What Your Doctor May Not Tell You About Menopause.* New York. Warner Books, 1996; 14

Massoudi, M.S., et. Al.—Prevalence of thyroid antibodies among healthy middle age women. Findings from the study in healthy women. *Annals of Epidemiology,* 1995; 5(3):229–233

Northrup, Christiane, M.D.—*The Wisdom of Menopause.* New York. Bantam Books, 2001; 111

Prestwood KM, Kenny AM, Unson C, Kulldorff M. The effect of low dose micronized 17b-estradiol on bone turnover, sex hormone levels, and side effects in older women: a randomized, double blind, placebo-controlled study. *Journal of Clinical Endocrinology and Metabolism* 2000 Dec;85(12):4462–9

Tzingounis VA, Aksu MF, Greenblatt RB. Estriol in the management of the menopause. *JAMA* 1978 Apr 21;239(16):1638–41.

Wilson, J.D.; Foster D.W.; Kronenberg, H.M.; and Larsen, P.R. eds. Williams *Textbook of Endocrinology* 9th Ed Philadelphia W.B. Saunders, 1998

Wright, J.V., M.D., and Morgenthaler, J.—*Natural Hormone Replacement;* CA, Smart Publications, 1997; 51

Zegura B, Keber I, Sebestjen M, Koenig W. Double blind, randomized study of estradiol replacement therapy on markers of inflammation, coagulation and fibrinolysis. *Atherosclerosis.* 2003 May;168(1):123–9.

Chapter 4

(2001). Testosterone Therapy: Spotlight On The Older Man At Last. *Health & Medicine Week.*

(2002). Hormone replacement therapy safe for most men with andropause. (In The Public Eye). *Urology Times,* 30(10), 16.

(2003). Male Menopause linked to higher risk of heart disease. *Heart Disease Weekly, 2.*

(2003). On Call—Hormone replacement therapy for men. (Letter to the Editor). *Harvard Men's Health Watch,* 7 (6).

(2003). Sexual dysfunction and andropause lead strong growth in men's segment. *Drug Week,* 279

(2004). Hormone therapy leads to high rates of osteoporosis in men. *Drug Week,* 411.

Carruthers, Malcom M.D., The Testosterone Revolution *Thorsons*

Channer, K.S., & Jones, T.H.,—Cardiovascular effects of testosterone: implications of the 'male menopause'? (Editorial) *Heart,* 2003; 89(2):121–123.

CMP Information Ltd. (2004). Is there a male menopause and should we treat it? **Puke,** 62.

Cutler, B.—Marketing to menopausal men *American Demographics* 1993; 15(3):49

Gray A, Feldman HA, McKinlay JB, Longcope C.—Age disease, and changing sex hormone levels in middle-aged men: results of the

Massachusetts Male Aging Study. *J Clin Endocrnol Metab* 1991; 73:1016–1025

Gould D.C., Petty R., & Jacobs H.S. (2000). The male menopause—does it exist? *British Medical Journal,* V320(7238), 858.

Groopman, J.—Hormones for Men. *The New Yorker.* 2002

Heller CG and Myers G.—The male climacteric, its symptomatology, diagnosis and treatment. *Journal of the American Medical Association* 1944; 126(8):472–477

Jenkins, T.—Male menopause: myth or monster? *Vibrant* L 1995; 11(6):12–15.

Kenny AM, Prestwood KM, Gruman CA, Marcello KM, Raisz LG—Effects of trandermal testosterone on bone and muscle in older men with low bioavailable testosterone levels. *Journals of Gerontology Series A: Biological Sciences and Medical Sciences.* 2001; 56(5)M266–72

Matsumoto AM,—Andropause: clinical implications of the decline in serum testosterone levels with aging in men. *Journals of Gerontology Series A: Biological Sciences and Medical Sciences*: 2002; 57(2): M76–99

Meagher, J.—Is male menopause just a myth? *Europe Intelligence Wire.* 2003

Morley JE.—Andropause, testosterone therapy and quality of life in aging men. *Cleveland Clinic Journal of Medicine* 2000; 67(12):880–2

Morley JE, Perry HM—Andropause: an old concept in new clothing. *Clinics in Geriatric Medicine* 2003; 19(3):507–528

Naish, J.—HRT for men? I don't believe it: is the male menopause fact or fiction? As John Naish reports, there is increasing controversy about treating men of certain age with testosterone. *Nursing Standard,* 2003; 17(37):202

Quallich, A.S.—Andropause. *Urologic Nursing,* 2003; 23(4):301302.

Rose, Marc R. MD, A Woman's Guide to Male Menopause—*Keats*

Sinclair J.F., Niederberger C.S. & Meacham R.B. (2003). Diagnosing androgen deficiency in the aging male. *Contemporary Urology,* 15(4), 70–75.

Shippen, Eugene MD, The Testosterone Syndrome—*Evans & Co.* 1988

Stas, SN, Anastasiadis AG, Fisch H, Benson MC, Shabsigh R.—Urologic aspects of andropause. *Urology* 2003; 61(2):261–6

Tan Rs—Andropause: introducing the concept of 'relative hypogonadism' in aging males. *International Journal of Impotence Research* 2002; 14(4):319

Tan Rs. Memory loss as a reported symptom of andropause.—*Arch of Androl* 2001;47:185–189

Tan Rs, Culberson JW—An integrative review on current evidence of testosterone replacement therapy for andropause. *Maturitas* 2003; 45(1):15–27

Tan R.S.; Philip P.S.—Perceptions of and Risk Factors for Andropause—*Archives of Andrologym* 1999 43(2,1):97–103(7)

Tan Rs, Pu SJ—Is it andropause? Recognizing androgen deficiency in aging men. *Postgraduate Medicine* 2004; 115(1):62–6

Tan Rs, Pu SJ.—The andropause and memory loss: is there a link between androgen decline and dementia in the aging male? *Asian J Androl* 2001;3:169–174

Tan Rs, Pu SJ, Culberson JW—Role of androgens in mild cognitive [thinking] impairment and possible interventions during andropause. *Medical Hypotheses* 2004; 62(1):14–8

Werner AA—The male climacteric: report of 273 cases. *Journal of the American Medical Association* 1946; 132:188–194

Ulrich, M.—Men who maunder about their fading virility should learn to grow old gracefully. *The Report Newsmagazine.* 2001

Urology Channel—Testosterone Deficiency

Wespes E, Schulmann CC.—Male andropause: myth, reality and treatment. *Int J Import Res* 2002; 14:S93–98

Chapter 5

Aldercreutz H. et al., Dietary Phyto-estrogens and the Menopause in Japan. *Lancet* 339:1233

Berkowitz Bob Ph.D., and Susan Yager-Berkowitz *He's Just Not Up for it Anymore*—HarperCollins Publishers 2008

Bernstein, L., C.R. Teal, S. Joslyn and J. Wilson Ethnicity-related variation in breast cancer risk factors.—*Cancer 97* 2003;1:222–229

Burkman R, Schlesselman JJ, Zieman M. Safety concerns and health benefits associated with oral contraception. *American Journal of Obstetrics and Gynecology* 2004; 190(4 Suppl):S5–22

Calcagni E, Elenkov I, Stress system activity, innate and T helper cytokines, and susceptibility to immune-related diseases. *Ann N Y Acad Sci* 2006; 1069:62–76

Cancer Prevention Coalition American Beef: Why is it banned in Europe?

Chen C. C., et al.—Adverse Life Events and Breast Cancer: Case-Control Study. *British Medical Journal* 1995; 311:1527–1530

Clemetson C.A.B., DeCarol S.J., Burney G.A., Patel T.J., Kozhiashvili N., et al.,—Estrogen in Food: The Almond Mystery. *International Journal of Gynecology and Obstetrics* 1978; 15:515–521

Collaborative Group on Hormonal Factors in Breast Cancer. Breast cancer and hormonal contraceptives: Collaborative reanalysis of individual data on 53,297 women with breast cancer and 100,239 women without breast cancer from 54 epidemiological studies. *Lancet* 1996; 347:1713–1727

Cornwall Warren and Keith Ervin "Hormonal chemicals may be imperiling fish"– *The Seattle Times*—2007

Cutter C.B., M.D.—Androgen Deficiency in Women: Understanding the Science, Controversy and Art of Treating our Patients—Part 1. *International Journal of Pharmaceutical Compounding,* 2004; S(1):16.

Diamond Jed *Surviving Male Menopause A Guide for Women and Men* 2000

Donovan, M., C. Tiwary, D. Axelrod, A. Sasco, L. Jones, R. Hajek, E. Sauber, J. Kuo, D. Davis Personal care products that contain estrogens or xenoestrogens may increase breast cancer risk.—*Medical Hypotheses* 68(4):756–766

Elakovich S.O., Hampton J.,—Analysis of Couvaestrol, A Phytoestrogen, in Alpha Tablest sold for Human Consumption. *Journal of Agricultural Food Chemistry* 1984; 32:173–175

Elenkov IJ, Chrousos GP—"Stress hormones, proinflammatory and anti-inflammatory cytokines, and autoimmunity." *Ann N Y Acad Sci* 2002; 966:290–303

Estrogens in personal care products. *Med Lett* 1985;27:54–5

Gandhi Renu PhD,BCERF Research Associate, Suzanne M. Snedeker, Ph.D., Research Project Leader, BCERF *Program on Breast Cancer and Environmental Risk Factors—Cornell University*—Consumer concerns about hormones in food—Fact Sheet #37: 2000

Giuca Linda, Nothing complex about choosing the right carbohydrates in diet. *The Milwaukee Journal Sentinel* 1999

Greer JB, Modugno F, Allen GO, Ness RB. Androgenic progestins in oral contraceptives and the risk of epithelial ovarian cancer. *Obstetrics and Gynecology* 2005; 105(4): 731–740

Goodwin Sarah, Stress affects hormones which affect immune system which alters mental and physical disease—*Medical News Today*—2004

Graham JD, Clarke CL. Physiological action of progesterone in target tissues. *Endocrine Reviews, 18,* 502–519.

Hertz R. Accidental ingestion of estrogens by children. *Pediatrics 21* 1958; p.203–206

Kershaw, Sarah Idahoans find cancers from fallout—4 Counties were exposed to high levels of radiation—*The New York Times* 2004 p.14

Lee John R. & Virginia Hopkins "Part II: Xenohormones in your environment. Rounding up the usual suspects when it come to chemicals, assume the worst and when in doubt, don't."—*John R. Lee Medical Letter*

Marchbanks PA, McDonald JA, Wilson HG et al "Oral contraceptives and the risk of breast cancer"—*New England Journal of Medicine* 2002;346(26)2025–2032

Randall Madeleine Hormones and belly fat—*Overnights* 2004

Rowen, Robert Jay, MD—Redesigned supplements fights breast and prostate cancer. 2005 15(8)

Schechter D. (1999). Estrogen, progesterone, and mood. *Journal of Gender Specific Medicine,* 1999; 2: 29–36.

Schildkraut JM, Calingaert B, Marchbanks PA, Moorman PG, Rodriguez GC. Impact of progestin and estrogen potency in oral contraceptives on ovarian cancer risk. *Journal of the National Cancer Institute* 2002; 94(1):32–38

Schuler Lou, Jeff Volek, R.D., PhD, Michael Mejia, and Adam Campbell *The Testosterone Advantage Plan Fireside* Publishers 2002

Schwarzman M, Potential toxicity of synthetic chemicals: What you should know about endocrine-disrupting chemicals.—*American Family Physician*—2008 78(5)

Shea, Katherine M., MD, Pediatric Exposure and Potential Toxicity of Phthalate Plasticizers" *MPH Pediatrics* 2003 111:1467–1474

Strauss, J.S., Hormones in personal care products. *JAMA* 1963 86:759–762

Ullis Karlis MD, *Super "T"*—Fireside 1999

U.S. Department of Health and Human Services, Public Health Service, National Toxicology Program Substance Profiles: Estrogens, Steroidal—*Report on Carcinogens,* Eleventh Edition 2005

Waldman, Peter, Presence of harmful chemicals in humans is broad common. *Wall Street Journal* 2005 p.B2

Wilsom, James l. (2001). *Adrenal Fatigue.* Smart Publications. Petaluma, CA

Wolff, M.S., J.A. Britton and V.P. Wilson Environmental risk factors for breast cancer among African-American women, *Cancer 97* 2003;1:289–310

Wright JV. (1999). Comparative measurements of serum estriol, estradiol, and E1 in non-pregnant, premenopausal women; A preliminary investigation. *Alternative Medicine Review, 4,* 266270.

Zimmerman, P.A., G.L. Fancis and M. Poth Hormone-containing personal care products may cause signs of early sexual development.—*Mil Med 160* 1995;p.628–630

Chapter 6

Allan, C.A. & McLachan, R.I. Age-related changes in testosterone and the role of replacement therapy in older men. *Clinical Endocrinology* 2004; 60:653–670

Araujo, A.B., O'Donnell, A.B., Brambilla, D.J., Simpson, W.D., Longcope, C., Matsumoto, A.M., et al. Prevalence and incidence of androgen deficiency in middle-age and older men: Estimates from the NMAS. *Journal of Clinical Endocrinology and Metabolism* 2004'89(12)5920–5926

Aversa, A., Isidors, A.M., Spera, G., ,Lenzi, A., & Fabbri, A. Androgens improve vasodilatation and response to slidenafil and patients with erectile dysfunction. Clinical Endocrinology, 2003;58(5) 632–638

Bagatell, C.J., & Bremner, W.J. Androgen and progestagen effects on plasma lipids. *Progress in Cardiovascular Diseases* 1995;38(3):255–271

Balkau Beverley, PhD; John E. Deanfield, MD, FRCP; Jean-Pierre Despres, PhD; jean-Pierre Bassand, MD, FESC; Deith A.A. Fox, FESC; Sidney C. Smith, Jr, MD; Philip Barter, MBBS, PhD; Chee-Eng Tan, MD, PhD; Luc Van Gaal, MD PhD; Hans-Ulrich Wittchen, PhD; Christine Massien, MD; Steven M. Haffner, MD International Day for the Evaluation of Abdominal Obesity (IDEA)—A Study o f Waist Circumference, Cardiovascular Disease, and Diabetes Mellitus in 168 000 Primary Care Patients in 63 Countries– *The American Heart Association* 2007;116:1942–1951

Braverman Eric, MD Reverse Aging by Restoring Youthful Sexual Function—*Life Extension Magazine* 2008

Davis, William MD. The Intimate Link Between Erectile Dysfunction and Heart Disease—*Life Extension Magazine* 2007

Dhindsa, S., Prabhakar, S., Sethi, M. Bandyopadhyay, A., Chaudhuri, A., & Dandona, P. Frequent occurrence of hypogonadotropic hypogonadism in type 2 diabetes. *Journal of clinical Endocrinology & Metabolism* 2004;89(11):5462–5468

Freeman, E.R., Bloom, D.A., & McGuire, E.J. A brief history of testosterone. *Journal o f Urology* 2001;165(2):371–373

Hu Gang, MD, PhD; Jaakko Tuomilehto, MD, PhD; Karri Silventoinen, PhD; Cinzia Sarti, MD, PhD; Satu Mannisoto, PhD; Pekka Jousilahti, MD, PhD—Body mass Index, Waist Circumference, and Waist-Hip Ration on the Risk of Total and Type-Specific Stroke—*Internal Medicine* 2007; 164(13):1420–1427

Institute of Medicine (IOM) Testosterone and aging: Clinical research directions *Washington D.C. IOM* 2003

Jankowska Eewa A., MD, Phd; Bartosz Biel, MD; Jocek Majda, PhD; Alicja Szklarska, PhD; Stefan D. Anker, MD, PhD; Waldemar

Banasiak, MD, PhD; Phlip A. Poole –Wilson, MD, FRCP; Piotr Ponikowski, MD, PhD Anabolic Deficiency in Men with Chronic Heart Failure—Prevalence and Detrimental Impact on Survival—*The American Heart Association*, 2006; 114:1829–1837

Key T, Appleby P, Barnes I, Reeves G; Endogenous Hormones and Breast Cancer Collaborative Group.—Endogenous sex hormones and breast cancer in postmenopausal women: reanalysis of nine prospective studies. *J Natl Cancer Ins*. 2002; 94(8):606–16

Khaw Kay-Tee, Mitch Dowsett, Elizabeth Folkerd, Sheila Bingham, Nicholas Wareham, Robert Luben, Ailsa Welch and Nicholas Day Endogenous Testosterone and mortality Due to all Causes, Cardiovascular Disease, and Cancer in Men: European Prospective Investigation into Cancer in Norfolk (EPIC-Norfolk) Prospective Population Study.—*The American Heart Association* 2007; 116: 2694–2707

Lee John R, MD *Hormone Balance for Men, What our Doctor May Not Tell You about Prostate Health and Natural Hormone Supplementation*—2003

Navar Paul, MD—Optimizing Testosterone levels in Aging Men *Life Extension Magazine* 2008

Pattarozzi Alessandra, Monica Gatti, Federica Barbieri, Roberto Wurth, Carola Porcile, Gianluigi Lunardi, Alessandra Ratto, Roberto Favoni, Adriana Bajetto, Angelo Ferrari, and Tullio Florio—17B—Estradiol Promotes Breast cancer Cell Proliferation –Inducing Stromal Cell-Derived Factor—1—Mediated Epidermal Growth Factor Receptor Transactivation: Reverasl By Gefitinib Pretreatment Molecular *Pharmacology Fast Forward* 2007; 10.1124/mol.107.039974

Reuters Health—Large waistlines associated with stroke risk—*Stroke* 2008

Rock Cheryl L., Shirley w. Flatt, Gail A. Laughlin, Ellen B. Gold, Cynthia A. Thomson, Loki Natarajan, Lovell A. Jones, Bette J. Caan,

Marcia L. Stefanick, Richard A. Hajek, Wael K. Al-Delaimy, Frank Z. Stanczyk, and John P. Pierce Reproductive Steroid Hormones and Recurrence-Free Survival in Women with a History of Breast Cancer—*Epidemiology Biomarkers & Prevention* 2008 17:614–620

Seidman SN—Testosterone deficiency and mood in aging men: pathogenic and therapeutic interactions. *World J Bio Psychiatry* 2003;4(1): 14–20

Whitmer R.A., D.R. Gustafson, E. Barrett-Connor, M.N.Haan, E.P. Gunderson and K. Yaffe Central obesity and increased risk of dementia more than three decades later"—*Neurology*, 2008; 71:1057–1064

Womens Health Initiative—WHI Follow up Study Confirms Health Risks of Long-Term Combination Hormone Therapy Outweigh Benefits for Postmenopausal Women—*U.S. Department of Health and Human Services NIH News National Institutes of Health* 2008

Zhang Cuilin, MD, PhD; Kathryn M. Rexrode, MD, MPH; Rob M. van Dam,, PhD; Tricia Y. Li, MD, MS; Frank B. Hu, MD, Phd Abdominal Obesity and the Risk of All-Cause Cardiovascular, and Cancer Mortality; Sixteen Years of Follow-up in US Women—*The American Heart Association* 2008;117:1658–1667

Chapter 7

Bachman, D.L.—Sleep Disorders with Aging: Evaluation and Treatment. *Geriatrics* 1992; 47(9):53–61

Bachmann G.A., et al.—Female Sexuality During the Menopause. *OBG Management suppl.* 1999 11(5)

Bales L.—Treatment of the Perimenopausal Female. *Primary Care Update Ob/Gyns* 1998; 5(2):90–94

Bonnick S.L., Johnson C.C. Jr., Kleerekoper M., et al.—Importance of precision in bone density measurements. *Journal of Clinical Densitometry,* 2001; 105–110

Campagnoli C, Abba C, Ambroggio S, Peris C. Pregnancy, progesterone and progestins in relation to breast cancer risk. *J Steroid Biochem Mol Biol* 2005; 97(5):441–50

Cauley J.A., Lucas F.L., Kuller L.H., et al.—Bone Mineral Density and Risk of Breast Cancer in Older Women: The Study of Osteoporotic Fractures. *The Journal of the American Medical Association* 1996; 276:1404

Chang KJ et al. Influences of percutaneous administration of estradiol and progesterone on human breast epithelial cycle in vivo. *Fertility and Sterility* 1995; 63:785–91

Clardson T.B.—The Effects of Hormone Replacement Therapy on Key Factors for Cardiovascular Disease. *Hormone Replacement Therapy Cardiovascular Health.* Fairlawn, NJ: MPE Communications. 2000

Cowan LD et al. Breast cancer incidence in women with a history of progesterone deficiency. *American Journal of Epidemiology* 1981; 114:209–17

Cummings S.R., Black D.M., Rubin S.M.—Lifetime risk of hip. Colles: or vertebral fracture and coronary heart disease among white postmenopausal women. *Archives of Internal Medicine, 1989; 14:* 2445–2448

Dalton K. The Premenstrual Syndrome and Progesterone Therapy. London, England: *William Heinemann* 1984

Dennerstein L., et al.—Sexuality, hormones and the menopause transition. *Maturitas* 1979; 26:83–93

DeSouzaM.J., Prestwood K.M., Luciano A.A., Miller B.E., Nulsen J.C.—A Comparison of the Effect of Synthetic and Micronized Hormone Replacement Therapy on Bone Mineral Density and Biochemical Markers of Bone Metabolism. *Journal of the North American Menopausal Society 1996; 3:*140

Desreux J, Kebers F, Noel A, Francart D, Van Cauwenberge H, Heinen V, Thomas JL, Bernard AM, Paris J, Delansorne R, Foidart JM. Progesterone receptor activation– an alternative to SERMs in breast cancer. *Eur J Cancer* 2000; 36(4):S90–1

Dören M, Nilsson J-A, Johnell O. Effects of specific post-menopausal hormone therapies on bone mineral density in post-menopausal women: a meta-analysis. *Human Reprod* 2003; 18(8):1737–1746

Effects of Oral and Transdermal Hormone Replacement Therapies on Serum Lipid and Lipoprotein Concentrations. *Obstetrics and Gynecology, 84*:222

Facts on Osteoporosis and Related Bone Diseases.—*National Resource Center, National Institutes of Health, Bethesda, MD.* 2002

Faulkner K.G., von Stecten E., Miller P.—Discordance in patient classification using T-scores. *Journal of Clinical Densitometry* 1999; 2:343–350

Fitzpatrick Lorraine A., Cindy Pace, Brinda Wiita. Comparison of Regimens Containing Oral Micronized Progesterone or Medroxyprogesterone Acetate on Quality of Life in Postmenopausal Women: *A Cross-Sectional Survey Journal of Women's Health & Gender-Based Medicine* 2000; 9(4): 381–387

Fournier A, Berrino F, Riboli E, Avenel V, Clavel-Chapelon F. Breast cancer risk in relation to different types of hormone replacement therapy in the E3N-EPIC cohort. *International Journal of Cancer* 2005; 114:448–454

Fox N.F., Chan J.K., Tharner M, et al.—Medical expenditures for the treatment of osteoporosis fractures in the United States in 1995: Report from the National Osteoporosis Foundation. *Journal of Bone and Mineral Research, 1997; 12*:24–35

Gallagher J.C., Rapuri P.B., Haynatzki G., Detter J.R.—Effect of discontinuation of estrogen calcitriol, and the combination of both on bone density and bone markers. *Journal of Clinical Endocrinology & Metabolis* 2002; *87*:4914–4923

Gilson G.R. M.D., Ph.D., Zava D.T.,PhD.—A Perspective on HRT for Women: Picking Up The Pieces After the Women's Health Initiative Trial, Part 2. *International Journal of Pharmaceutical Compounding, 2002; 7(5),* 330–338

Hargrove JT, Maxson WS, Wentz AC, Burnett LS. Menopausal hormone replacement therapy with continuous daily oral micronized estradiol and progesterone. *Obstet Gynecol* 1989; 73:606–612

Heart Disease Is The Number 1 Killer of Women in the United States. *Heart Strong Women. The American College of Obstetricians and Gynecologists.* 1998

Holt, Stephen. M.D.—The Antiporosis Plan: A Wellness Guide. *Wellness Publishing.* 2002

Jones NC, Constantin D, Prior MJ, et al. *European Journal of Neuroscience* 2005; 21(6):1547

Kaaks R, Berrino F, Key T, Rinaldi S, Dossus L, Biessy C, Secreto G, Amiano P, Bingham S, Boeing H, Bueno de Mesquita HB, Chang-Claude J, Clavel-Chapelon F, Fournier A, van Gils CH, Gonzalez CA, Barricarte Gurrea A, Critselis E, Khaw KT, Krogh V, Lahmann PH, Nagel G, Olsen A, Onland-Moret NC, Overvad K, Palli D, Panico S, Peeters P, Quirós JR, Roddam A, Thiebaut A, Tjønneland A, Chirlaque MD, Trichopoulou A, Trichopoulos D, Tumino R, Vineis P, Norat T, Ferrari P, Slimani N, Riboli E. Serum sex steroids in premenopausal women and breast cancer risk within the European Prospective Investigation into Cancer and Nutrition (EPIC). *J Natl Cancer Inst* 2005; 97:755–65

Kanis J.A., for the WHO study group.—Assessment of fracture risk and its application to screening for postmenopausal osteoporosis: synopsis of a WHO report. *Osteoporosis International* 1994; 4:368–361

Koefoed P., Brahm J.—The permeability of the human red cell membrane to steroid sex hormones. *Biochimica et Biophysics Acta,* 1994; 1195:55–62

Laidlaw IJ, Clarke RB. The proliferation of normal cell tissue implanted into athymic nude mice is stimulated by estrogen, but not by progesterone. *Endocrinology* 1995; 136: 164–71

Lee JR. Osteoporosis reversal; the role of progesterone. *International Clinical Nutrition Review* 1990; 10(3):384–91

Lee JR. Is natural progesterone the missing link in osteoporosis prevention and treatment? *Med Hypotheses* 1991; 35:316–318

Lee JR. Osteoporosis reversal with transdermal progesterone. *Lancet* 1990; 336:1327

Leonetti H., M.D., Longo S., M.D., Anasti J., M.D. (1999)

Liang M, Liao EY, Xu X, Luo XH, Xiao XH. Effects of progesterone and 18-methyl levonorgestrel on osteoblastic cells. *Endocr Res* 2003; 29(4):483–501

Lindsay R.—Prevention and Treatment of Osteoporosis. *Lancet* 1993; 341:801

Marshall D., Johnell Q., Wedel H.—Meta-analysis of how well measures of bone mineral density predict occurrence of osteoporotic fractures. *British Medical Journal,* 1996; 372:1254–1259

Maxson WS. The use of progesterone in the treatment of PMS. *Clin Obstet Gynecol.* 1987; 30:465–477

Molinari C, Battaglia A, Grossini E et al.—"Effect of progesterone on peripheral blood flow in prepubertal female anesthetized pigs." *Journal of Vascular Research.* 2001; 38:569–577

Newton K.M., LaCroix A.Z.—Hormone Replacement Therapy and Tertiary Prevention of Coronary Heart Disease. *Menopausal Medicine* 1999; 7(2):5–8

NIH Consensus Development Panel.—Osteoporosis Prevention, Diagnosis, and Therapy. *The Journal of the American Medical Association* 2001; 285:785

Noteloviz Morris, M.D., Ph.D., *Stand Tall: Every Woman's Guide to Preventing and Treating Osteoporosis* Triad Publishing Company 1998

Plu-Bureau G, Le MG, Thalabard JC, Sitruk-Ware R, Mauvais-Jarvis P. Percutaneous progesterone use and risk of breast cancer: results from a French cohort study of premenopausal women with benign breast disease. *Cancer Detect Prev* 1999; 23(4):290–6

Prestwood K.M., Kenny A.M., Kleppinger A., Kulldorff M.—Ultralow-Dose Micronized 17-Estradiol and Bone Density and Bone Metabolism in Older Women: A Randomized Controlled Trial The journal *of the American Medical Association* 2003; 290,10421048

Prior JC, Vigna Y, Alojado N. Progesterone and the prevention of osteoporosis. *Canadian Journal of Obstetrics/Gynecology and Women's Health Care* 1991; 3(4):178–84

Prior JC, Vigna YM, Schecter MI, Burgess AE. Spinal bone loss and ovulatory disturbances. *New England Journal of Medicine* 1990; 323(18):1221–7

Prior JC. Progesterone as a bone-trophic hormone. *Endocr Rev* 1990; 11(2):386–98

Randolph C.W. Jr. M.D., *Natural Hormone Balance* Women's Medicine, Inc. 1999

Rosano G.M., Webb C.M., Chierchia S et al.—Natural progesterone, but not medroxyprogesterone acetate, enhances the beneficial effect of estrogen on exercise-induced myocardial ischemia in postmenopausal women. *Journal of the American College of Cardiology, 2000;* 36:2154–2159

Schwartz E., M.D.—*The Hormone Solution.* New York: Warner Books 2002

Sherwin B.B.—Estrogen Effects of Cognition on Menopausal Women. *Neurology 48 suppl,* 1997; S21–S26

Siris E.S., Miller P.D., Barrett-Connor E., et al.—Identification and fracture outcomes of undiagnosed low bone mineral density in postmenopausal women: results from the National Osteoporosis Risk Assessment. *The Journal of the American Medical Association, 2001;* 286:2815–2822

Sotelo M., Johnson S.R.—The Effects of Hormone Replacement Therapy on Coronary Heart Disease. *Endocrinology and Metabolism Clinics of North America* 1997; 26(2):313–327

Sowers M, Randolph JF Jr, Crutchfield M, Jannausch ML, Shapiro B, Zhang B, La Pietra M. Urinary ovarian and gonadotropin hormone levels in premenopausal women with low bone mass. *J Bone Miner Res* 1998; 13(7):1191–202

Speroff L.—Hormone Replacement Therapy: Clarifying the Picture. *Hospital Practice.* 2001 www.hosppract.com/issues/2001/05/dmm spe.htm

Speroff L.—Postmenopausal Hormone Therapy and Cardiovascular System. Oregon Health Services University School of Medicine. *Contemporary Ob/Gyn,* 1997; 426

Speroff L.—The Heart and Estrogen/Progestin Replacement Study (HERS). *Maturitas,* 1998; 31(3): 9

Spiegel K, Leproult R, Van Cauter E.—Impact of Sleep Debt in Metabolic and Endocrine Function. *Lancet* 1999; 354:1435–1439

Stein DG, *Brains Res Rev* 2008; 57(2):3860397

Stein DB, Wright DW, Kellerman, *AL. Annuals of Emergency Medicine* 2008; 51(2):164–172

Stephenson K, Neuenschwander PF, Kurdowska AK, Pinson B, Price C. Transdermal Progesterone Effects on Menopausal Symptoms and on Thrombotic, Anticoagulant, and Inflammatory Factors in Postmenopausal Women. *International Journal of Pharmaceutical Compounding,* 2008; 12(4): 295–304

Taskinen M.R., et al.—Hormone Replacement Therapy Lowers Plasma Lp(a) Concentrations, Comparison Cyclic Transdermal and Continuous Estrogen Progestin Regimens. *Arteriosclerosis, Thrombosis, and Vascular Biology,* 1996; 16:1215–1221

Transdermal Progesterone Cream for Vasomotor Symptoms and Postmenopausal Bone Loss. *Obstetrics and Gynecology* 1994; 2:225–228

Washburn S.A.—Estradiol and Progesterone Effects on the Central Nervous System. *Menopausal Medicine* 1997; *5(4):5–8*

Waddell B.J., Leary P.C.O.—Distribution and metabolism of topically applied progesterone in a rat model. *Journal of Steroid Biochemistry and Molecular Biology,* 2001; *80:*449–455

Whitcroft S.I., Crook D, Marsh M.S., et al.—Long Term 1994

Williams JK, Honore EK, Washburn SA et al. (1994). "Effects of hormone replacement therapy on reactivity of artherosclerotic coronary arteries in cynomolgus monkeys." *Journal of American College of Cardiology.* 1994; 224:1757–1761

Writing Group for the Women's Health Initiative.—Risks and benefits of estrogen plus progestin in health menopausal women. *The Journal of the American Medical Association,* 2002*;* 288*:*321–333

Zhang Y., et al. (1998). Bone Mass and the Risk of Cancer Among Postmenopausal Women. *New England Journal of Medicine,* 1998; 336: 611–617

Index

Page numbers followed by an *f* or *t* indicate figures or tables.